SICK NOTES

True Stories from
the Front Lines of Medicine

Tony Copperfield

Monday Books

A CIP catalogue record for this title is available
from the British Library

ISBN: 978-1-906308-14-8

Typeset by Andrew Searle
Printed and bound by Cox and Wyman

www.mondaybooks.com
http://mondaybooks.blogspot.com/
info@mondaybooks.com

Dr Tony Copperfield is the pseudonymous creation of two practising GPs. To preserve patient confidentiality, none of the characters in the book exist, but the opinions expressed are real, allowing for some comic exaggeration, and the events are all based on truth or actually happened. Together, they paint a very accurate picture of life in general practice. Trust us, we're doctors.

Dr. Tony Copperfield is the pseudonymous creation of two practising GPs. To preserve patient confidentiality none of the characters in the book exist, but the opinions expressed are real, although for some comic example, and the or part are all based on truth or actually happened. Together they paint a very accurate picture of life in general practice. Trust me, we're doctors.

THE DOCTOR WILL SEE YOU NOW

MY NAME'S DR TONY COPPERFIELD, and I'm a general practitioner.

There! Got that off my chest.

If it sounds like I'm at a Medics Anonymous meeting, confessing to vocation addiction, nothing could be further from the truth: some days I could give up general practice just like that… no withdrawal symptoms, no 'taking each day as it comes', no sneaky blood pressure checks when no one's looking.

In fact, hanging up my stethoscope would be very easy indeed.

Particularly on one of those days when I arrive to find that the practice computers have crashed, or one of my partners is off sick, or the flu season is kicking in, or the slimeball TV doctor this morning covered his/her backside by suffixing every piece of advice with, 'If you're really worried, see your GP', or the switchboard's on meltdown, or the visit book's on to its third page by 9.30am, or my first three patients each bring a list because, 'I don't come very often, doctor,' or there are no biscuits or coffee but there are a lot of 'extras' at the end of morning surgery, or I'm constantly interrupted by phone calls from the distressed, deranged or dysfunctional, or my pigeon hole's bulimic with paperwork, or I'm already late for the first of three meetings and I may not be feeling too well myself because, amazingly, GPs have a psyche and a soma too, and both may be suffering from last night's therapeutic dose of cabernet sauvignon.

Other days are just fine.

So I guess it's like any other job, except that the key aspects are perhaps more amplified: the frustration, the satisfaction, the distraction, the rewards and – always lurking, ready to stab you in the back – the potential for disaster.

One way of training for this would be to try to do the *Times* crossword on a high wire while one person shouts at you and another hits you with a plank. Instead, we use a decade of medical school and postgraduate training. There are about 41,000 of us. Mostly, we operate in practices, which are businesses contracted by the local Primary Care Trust (PCT). Mine, consisting of five full time ('whole time equivalent') GPs, is pretty typical, but there's quite a range, from single-handers working in splendid isolation to huge conglomerates which could be mistaken for a small hospital.

We GPs are, in the main, self-employed, but we need some organising – plus there are reception staff, nurses and the like to employ, rotas to sort, meetings to arrange, complaints to deal with, health and safety to cackle over and so on. That's why virtually every practice has a manager – he or she can drown in paperwork and bureaucracy while we docs see patients… and also drown in paperwork and bureaucracy.

Pay is a hot topic at the moment. Yes, we're rewarded well, but for the vast majority of GPs the figures bear no resemblance to those amusing headlines in the papers. Some workaholics squeeze serious money out of the system; for most of us, the salary reflects the time we spend training and the responsibilities we take on. *How* we're paid is unbelievably complex and it changes every five minutes. Later, I'll try to explain it though, like many other GPs, I don't fully understand it myself.

So what about the job itself? We're contracted to provide family doctor services from 8am to 6.30pm, though the government has recently bullied us into providing 'extended hours' surgeries in the evenings and weekends for those too busy to be ill at conventional times. We also do some home visits – hence the 'visit book' above; urgent visits are done pronto by the duty doc, the others are divvied up amongst us after surgery. Anything outside the 8am to 6.30pm and extended hours slots comprises 'Out-of-hours', which is also 'out-of-my-control'. When, some years ago, our revised contract relieved GPs of the considerable burden that was out-of-hours, there was much chucking of hats in the air – none higher than mine, as it was the bane of my life, and now it's the PCT's problem.

Each GP has around 2,000 patients to look after, and we're the first port of call for whatever symptom you might dream up (if you ignore pharmacists, that is – and we try to, given some of the stuff they peddle). If it's an emergency – a very wide definition – we'll see you ASAP, and if you want a standard appointment it'll usually be within 48 hours if you don't mind who you see (you guessed, a government target). Otherwise, it's pot luck and can be anything from same day to a couple of weeks depending on holidays, epidemics, popularity of doctor and so on.

Though we might appear cynical, we GPs are actually quite proud of our role – particularly the 'gate-keeping' part. Here's how it works. The GP's knowledge is very broad but superficial, as opposed to the specialist's, which is narrow but deep. (If you prefer, GPs know something about everything while specialists know everything about something.) Combine these two skill-sets and you have an excellent system. GPs filter out the vast masses of 'worried well', only allowing through the hospital gates the few who really do need a good poking with a colonoscope. Patients are saved from unnecessary – sometimes dangerous – tests, and hospitals are saved from unnecessary patients. It's a safe, sensible and very efficient approach.

There's more to the job than that, though. We're also experts at creating order from chaos. Patients often present multiple problems, in confusing ways, plus we have the disadvantage of seeing illness at its earliest and most perplexing stages. Factor in large dollops of patient anxiety, the usual, 'While I'm here, doctor' extra agenda, our role as confidante and health co-ordinator together with the distraction of junior trying to pull the electricity cable out of my computer and you start to appreciate that general practice is as much art as science.

Which is why we GPs view the Great and Good – who dish out guidelines based on clear cut, text-book cases and subscribe to a tick-box culture of measuring only what can easily be measured – with great scepticism. In fact, we view most individuals who aren't GPs with great scepticism, because you really need to have done it to truly appreciate it.

There are times when it goes swimmingly. And there are times when it goes pear-shaped. And in those dark days, it feels like the myriad agencies we interact with – the hospital doctors, district nurses, social workers, health visitors, the academics, the bureaucrats at the PCT, even the receptionists (Gawd bless 'em) and, it has to be said, the patients – *especially* the patients – conspire to make a tricky job nigh on impossible.

So it's not something you'd get addicted to, though you get used to the taste after a while.

My name's Tony Copperfield, and welcome to my world.

HELL IS OTHER PEOPLE'S VOMIT

DESPITE THE ABOVE moan, I wouldn't swap what I do for anything. But Monday mornings are still hell, and the first Monday morning of the new year is hell squared, so it was with a sinking feeling that I nosed my car into the Senior Partner's space the other day. (I'm not actually the Senior Partner; I just like to live life on the edge.)

Bleak House practice is located at one end of a small shopping centre which is itself on the outskirts of a sprawling estate of beige, shoebox houses. The view from my window is of a branch of Spar.

Next to that is Bargain Booze, next to *that* is a 99p store and the rest of the row is made up of chippies, charity shops and a pharmacy.

In keeping with the locale, our building is a squat grey monstrosity. It's owned by the Primary Care Trust, which is, naturally, based in a gleaming new HQ which cost untold millions and looks like something out of *Battlestar Galactica*. By contrast, our rat hole positively reeks of decay. It was designed in the 1960s, built in the 1970s, remodelled for disabled access in the 1990s and has been scheduled for demolition and replacement ever since. When – or perhaps if, given the state of the economy – the new one is eventually built, it would be nice if it was more health centre and less concrete cancer.

I paused before opening the reception door. On the bricks above the portico, someone had scrawled the words '*Fuck you knobhead*'. I'm not sure why, but this piece of graffito seemed to me to be the perfect mission statement for us. It certainly beats 'Working in the community for your good health'. I resolved to suggest we add it to our headed notepaper at the next Partners' Meeting.

I pushed open the door and walked in.

It was only just 8am. The place was quiet, but the atmosphere was pregnant with anticipation – like a Caribbean island awaiting a hurricane, or a battlefield before the first shots are fired. Within half an hour, chaos would reign: standing room only, phones ringing off the hook, a dozen overweight mums pushing buggies back and forward and a gaggle of confused and apprehensive elderly people huddling in a corner as snotty-nosed toddlers hurtle around, shrieking. But for now, there was only a scattering of early birds. A teenaged girl and her worried mother sat together glumly, the girl flicking desultorily through a dog-eared copy of *Heat*. A middle-aged male patient was jabbing his finger at a couple of nervous receptionists and snarling something about antibiotics. They used to be a bit less nervous in the days when they sat behind a thick plate glass screen, but that was removed a while ago after the PCT deemed it too 'threatening'. Lurking somewhere in the background, in case it got a bit tasty, was Mrs Peggotty, the reception manager. She hails from County Sligo, has a squint and forearms like an all-in wrestler, and she takes no nonsense from anyone.

There was only one other punter, an elderly man who was hovering near the desk, and he grabbed me on the sleeve as I passed.

'Here,' he said. 'Can you help me with this? Only I can't understand the bleeding thing.'

He was standing by the booking-in computer.

'Well,' I said. 'Where it says, *Enter date of birth*, you need to enter your date of birth.'

'Yerwhatter?' he said.

'What's your date of birth?' I said.

'July 11th, 1937. Only, it was the day George Gershwin died and...'

'Yes, yes,' I said. 'You see, you type that in here like *this*... and we find that you are Mr Alf Tupman of 15 Back Street. Do you see? And you have an appointment to see me at 8.40am. So it tells you to go and wait outside Room 3, which is my room. Is that OK?'

I hurried on before Mr Tupman could tell me, and the assembled throng, that the pile cream I had recently prescribed him was no bloody good.

DNA TESTS

MY FIRST PATIENT of the day was a 'DNA' – meaning she Did Not Attend.

You'd be surprised how many of these GPs get. The Royal College of General Practitioners says 10 million appointments a year end in a no-show. When you factor in that each appointment has a 10-minute slot set aside for it, you can see that literally years of quality doctoring time is being frittered away.

Officially, we think DNAs are a Very Bad Thing. From time to time, notices will appear in waiting rooms informing patients that 30 people failed to keep their appointments last Tuesday week, and that five hours of their doctor's precious time was wasted as a result. Some politicians have floated the idea of allowing us to charge non-attenders, while the more hard-hearted and money-grabbing members of my profession talk about charging *everyone* for appointments, on the basis that if they've paid for it they'll use it. (Opponents say that such charges might discourage patients from seeing the doctor. Er, yes. That's the whole idea.)

I suppose you do have to wonder exactly what kind of person might book an appointment to see a doctor, thus preventing anyone else from booking the same slot, and then not bother to show up, but the fact is – entirely *un*officially – I love DNAs.

As I sat there at my desk, contemplating a mound of unopened and almost certainly pointless post from the previous Friday, Sami Patel popped his head round the door.

Sami, the most junior of our four partners, is a thrusting young lad from Manchester whose dad runs a big practice up there. He drives a silver Porsche Boxter, his girlfriend looks like Miss India's prettier sister and he is a very good doctor. I ought to hate him, but somehow I just can't.

'I thought you were off today,' I said.

'I am,' he said. 'I've just nipped in to get my QOF points in order.'

Sami is mad about QOF – Quality and Outcomes Framework – points, of which more later.

'Anyway,' he went on, 'you'll love this, Copperfield. Bloody Gordon in reception obviously forgot I was off, because he's just put a call through to me from a bloke who was due in for his well-person check on Friday when he twisted his ankle on the way. So he limps off to A&E, where they fob him off with a script for some anti-inflammatories, which obviously he's got to pay for, and he rings up this morning to apologise for not coming in. So I say to him, "You had to pay for your ibuprofen, you had to fork out six quid to park there and now the the Health Select Committee is talking about fining you for missing his GP appointment. Your ankle may not be broke, Mr Westlock, but you soon will be!" Get it? "Your ankle may not be broke…"'

'Very good, Sami,' I said. 'Stick the kettle on.'

Six quid to park at St George's, I thought. *Not to mention the fiver to pay some young scally to watch your car.* No wonder so many patients abuse the ambulance service: it's door-to-door, with no meter to feed. Gordon Brown promised to abolish car park charges at hospitals, but typically failed to suggest a realistic way of making up the resultant funding shortfall.

With six minutes to go before my next patient was due, I ambled down the corridor to the common room.

Sami was pouring boiling water into the cafetière.

'Hmmm,' I said, sniffing the air. 'Hand-roasted Guatemalan, if I'm not mistaken?'

He stopped stirring and stared at me. 'How did you…?'

'From Santa Ana la Huerta,' I said. 'Interlayered flavours, nuances of berries, honey and dark chocolate. A strong, yet elegant, bean.'

He followed my eyes to the packet of Union Hand Roasted Guatemala Coffee (100% Arabica, £2.79 from Ocado, tastes like the contents of a specimen jar) lying next to the kettle, and groaned.

He started pouring the coffee.

'What I said about DNAs,' he said. 'To be fair, the government has a point. You've had one first thing this morning, there was my

8

twisted ankle bloke on Friday, we had a dozen others that I can think of last week. We're averaging 60 a month, in this practice alone. It's tax-payers' money, is this. Personally, I agree – DNAs ought to be fined.'

'You must be mad,' I said. 'If we were to start fining them for not turning up, what do you think would happen?'

'Well,' he said, regarding me as though I were a simpleton. 'A few more of the buggers might turn up.'

'Precisely,' I said. 'Can you imagine what it would be like if everyone who booked an appointment at the surgery came in? When would we find the time to catch up on paperwork, check blood test results, write referrals? Not to mention coffee and Sudoku. The NHS would collapse overnight. Fine them? We should reward them.'

'Hmmm,' said Sami. 'I hadn't thought of it like that.'

'That makes two of you,' I said. 'You and the Secretary of State for Health.'

He meandered out, and I stood pondering awhile, safe in the knowledge that my own DNA afforded me a few minutes of precious peace, with nothing to concern me but a Hob Nob. If people don't want to turn up, that's their shout. I have far better things to do than checking Mr Harris's ankle jerks, trying to look at the tympanic membranes of malevolent three-year-olds and listening to Mrs Mowcher's description of her funny turns, the ones that only happen during *Coronation Street* on a Wednesday, for the 13th time to make sure I haven't missed an obvious diagnostic clue the first dozen times around. Give me a surgery of 17 booked appointments with 15 DNAs, and that's as near to heaven as I get.

TEN MINUTES

WE'RE SUPPOSED TO set aside 10 minutes for each consultation. It sounds a reasonable length of time, but there's a lot more to factor in than just the obvious. We can't physically eject patients while they're still talking, and we can't do much about those who turn up late and throw everything out of kilter. But even if every punter came in on time, sat down and spoke clearly and concisely about their precise symptoms for seven minutes, leaving me enough time to come up with a brilliant and incisive treatment strategy, or maybe just a quick prescription if I'm stretched, there'd still be calls to take from consultants, practice nurses and receptionists, hospital admissions to authorise, referrals to process, computer crashes and jammed printers to deal with, forms to fill in and QOF targets to hit.

The NHS's own online guidance to patients doesn't help. It advises them to turn up with 'a list of problems, starting with the most important'. 'If you have a complicated problem,' it says, 'ask for a longer appointment when you book… Be clear about what you want the doctor to do… Be assertive if you need to. Ask the doctor to repeat and explain anything you don't understand. If there are words you don't understand, ask what they mean or get the doctor to write them down so that you can look them up later.'

Which is all good advice to sensible folk like you and me and the people who wrote it, but in the real world not all patients are sensible. If a quarter of the people we see think they have complicated problems (when they haven't), bring a list and require – assertively – that we repeat, explain and write down anything they don't understand (i.e., everything), we'll need 30 minute slots and 36-hour days.

NEW YEAR, SAME STORY

WITH IT BEING January, I knew my surgeries would be filled with two types of bloke – each of them claiming they had decided to 'get healthy' in the New Year.

Mr Parkes fell into the first, more common category – those who have reluctantly decided that a diet of Quality Street, lager and Christmas pud, consumed while watching a loop of *The Great Escape*, is not the way forward.

Or – as in his case – have had this decided for them by their partner.

He'd brought Mrs Parkes with him, in the sense that a mouse brings a cat: it was clear his New Year's resolution had been thrust on him by his glowering wife, and he wore it forlornly, like an unwanted festive woolly.

'I'm a bit overweight,' he mumbled. 'I probably need more exercise and I should pack up the fags.'

'Tell him about your drinking,' prompted his other half, who had attended partly to hold his hand but mainly to make sure he didn't fluff his lines.

'I drink too much,' he said, like a teenager caught with a porn mag.

'And he can't…' said a voice from off-stage.

He turned crimson. 'And I can't… er… get it up.'

'That's right, doctor,' confirms Mrs Parkes. '*And* he has smelly feet.'

It's always tempting in these cases to suggest that the woman exchange her man for a sleeker, more vibrant, less pungent model. But I went through the motions and established that, yes, he was overweight, under-fit and led an unhealthy lifestyle. I gave him advice, unsurprisingly, about losing weight, dragging his ample arse down the gym and generally sorting himself out. Quite possibly he wasn't listening, but Mrs Parkes certainly was.

'Thanks, doctor,' she said as they left. Her husband and I simply exchanged glances. He'd done his duty, but we both knew that our next significant encounter might well be when I sign his cremation forms.

Mr Perker fell into the second category of January visitor.

'I've come for a check-up,' he announced.

Further inquiry revealed that he jogs 20 miles a week, eats the recommended quota of fruit and veg, is a non-smoker with perfect body-mass index, subscribes to *Men's Health* magazine and charts his own cholesterol and blood pressure stats on an Excel spreadsheet.

The truth was, he was only attending for positive reinforcement, like a class swot eager for the teacher to mark his homework.

Category two is far rarer than Category one – which is no bad thing because, while absurdly healthy, Perker's sort make me feel sick.

Both the seasonal polarities of male behaviour are the exceptions, though. For most men, January is just an arbitrary month on the calendar rather than a catalyst to a medical makeover. Maybe this is health negligence. Or perhaps it's a simple desire to avoid wasting time on imponderables. After all, exactly what is health? Don't expect the average doctor to provide an answer; we're paralysed with doubt just deciding whether sore throats need antibiotics*.

The World Health Organisation defines health as a 'state of complete physical, mental and social wellbeing and not merely the absence of disease'. This definition is, for practical purposes, useless. For the average male, it would mean celebrating a major lottery win with a dyspepsia-free curry and waking up to find that his scrotal lump is not cancer, that he has moved to Barbados and that Cindy

Crawford is downstairs cooking his brekkie. Oh, and that his team will stuff Man U eight-nil in the afternoon.

Besides, it sidesteps the issue that health is in the eye of the beholder.

Mr Parkes would make the man from WHO's toes curl, but may have happily reached his own limited personal physical, mental and social targets.

Mr Perker appears super-fit but has an unhealthy preoccupation with his own physiology.

So I'd suggest that health is feeling 'fit for a purpose', no matter how tiny or grand that purpose might be. Most blokes, I suspect, would accept this. Which means that they ought to spend January recovering from December, without having to make appointments they don't need and resolutions they won't keep.

*The answer to this question is usually No. Whether or not to prescribe antibiotics for sore throats (and if so, which ones to dish out and for how long) has been the subject of hundreds of clinical trials. At the moment, the best that we can manage is to follow a set of guidelines that tell us whether a prescription is more likely to help than harm the patient.

Of course there are more than one set of guidelines – in fact there are papers setting out guidelines on the use of guidelines – but most GPs will have heard of the 'Centor criteria'. On this scale, patients score one point if they have a fever, one point if they have tender swellings in the part of their neck under the chin, another point if there's a yellow gunky discharge over the tonsils and another point if they haven't got a cough. A score of zero has an 80% 'negative predictive value' – translated into English, if you have none of the above markers (but still have a sore throat), the chance of penicillin helping you is less than 20%. If you score three or four marks out of four, you have about a 50:50 chance of having a bacterial sore throat and you should be offered antibiotics. That doesn't mean you should take them. There are side-effects to taking antibiotics, and even if you score four points you'll get better without them; it's just that with them you might get better a day or so quicker.

TRUE COST OF DRUGS

JEFF BRICK was in to see me later on.

He never bloody listens to a word I say, which often leads me to wonder why he bothers consulting me. Mainly, I suspect, it's for his inhaler. After a lifetime working as an industrial welder on top of a 40-a-day Benson and Hedges habit, Jeff suffers, unsurprisingly, from dyspnoea (shortness of breath).

Periodically he comes in for a check-up and a new puffer, and I carefully explain the importance of using it properly, and taking exercise, and quitting the fags, and he nods blankly as the words enter his left ear and exit the right without troubling the scorers within.

Anyway, I printed off his prescription, signed it and handed it to him, and waited for him to get up and go. Instead, he sat there looking at it, his brow furrowed. Eventually, he said: 'What's this price thing by where it says about me inhaler, then?'

I took the script back. Sure enough, it was there in black and white. I read it out: 'Seretide 250 Evohaler. Use twice daily as directed. Supply 1 (one) inhaler. £59.48.'

'Hmmm,' I said. 'Well, for some reason I can't fathom, the computer has printed off the actual cost of the inhaler. It shouldn't do, and as I say I'm not sure why it has, but there it is. That's what they cost – nearly sixty quid.'

'You're taking the piss, mate,' he said. 'I ain't payin' that.'

'You're not,' I said. 'It's just the usual seven quid-odd to you. The £59.48 is what it costs the NHS.'

'You're 'avin' a larf!'

'Er, no.'

'You're pullin' my plonker!'

'Look… no, I'm not. That really *is* what the NHS spends on the inhalers which you use like air fresheners because you can't be bothered to read the instructions.'

'Stone me.'

I'd quite like to, I thought, as he shambled out, muttering to himself.

I called through to reception. 'For some reason, my PC is printing scripts off with the prices,' I said.

'Yes,' said Mrs Peggotty, the reception manager. 'I've just had Dr Emma call me to say the same thing. I'm ringing the IT people now doctor, don't you worry.'

The NHS IT infrastructure which helps me 'Deal With Today's Problems Today!'®, runs on vastly outdated software, so perhaps I ought to be thankful that it only crashes and burns every other fortnight. Still, it won't surprise any reader with half an interest in government computer systems to learn that this particular problem persisted for a further five days.

I say 'problem', but it was actually a blessing. In fact, it was brilliant and it ought to be a permanent feature of all prescriptions and medicine labels: if patients knew the real cost of their medication, maybe they'd be less cavalier about forgetting to take it, losing it or flushing it down the loo. Those who pay prescription charges and bitch about forking out £7.20 per item – pretty cheap for an inhaler costing nearly 60 quid – might change their tune, as would those who buy an annual ticket for £104 and act as though they're taking out a second mortgage, rather than handing over the price of a second-hand Nintendo Wii.

Conversations along similar lines peppered the next few days. Psoriasis sufferers couldn't believe a month's supply of scalp ointment ran to £108, a man on anticonvulsants had a fit – well, nearly – when he realised how much he was denting the NHS budget, and an old lady taking a cholesterol-lowering drug actually apologised when she found out that she was costing the NHS £80 every time she handed in her repeat prescription on the first of the month. And *she* was one of the ones where the money seemed well spent (I'm afraid that making value judgments about my patients goes with the territory).

So by the time Yvonne Claypole rang I was well up for it.

'Hello doc, listen, do me a favour, yeah?' she said. 'Only, I went over to Bristol to see my sister's family at the weekend, yeah? I had the prescription you gave me last week for my migraines made up while I was there, yeah, and, d'you know what, I've only gone and left all me tablets down there. Leave another prescription with Mrs Peggotty in reception, there's a love, and I'll pick it up in the morning.'

'Can you just hang on a mo?' I said. 'I just want to check something.'

I laid the receiver down, printed a script off and looked at it.

Imigran Radis tablets 100mg. Take one at onset of migraine. Supply 1 (one) pack of 12 (twelve) tablets. £85.80.

Eighty. Five. Quid. On headache tablets for a woman who is so bothered about her problem that she has forgotten where she put the last lot of pills.

I got on to Google. Then I picked the phone back up.

'Listen, Yvonne,' I said. 'Can you get yourself to the coach station in town by 8pm? There's a bus to Bristol leaving at half past. It's £18.50 return. And do give my best wishes to your sister and her family.'

DRUG BUDGETS

GIVEN THE ABOVE, I suppose I ought to explain drug budgets. We don't have one, as such – in the sense that you can't run out of money, come November. What we do have is an Indicative Prescribing Budget (IPB) and a Prescribing Incentives Scheme (PIS).

The IPB was introduced a while back and is an amount of money allocated to your practice on a computer at the PCT. It's based on the number of patients on your list, some very basic and unsophisticated demographics (a GP in Eastbourne might get a little more money to reflect the fact that all his punters are OAPs), and also on historical prescribing patterns. (In the months before it came in, I'm told that some unscrupulous doctors were wildly prescribing everything they could to anyone they found near the surgery, on the basis that this would push their budget up. A nice idea – wish I'd thought of it.)

The incentives scheme is a list of criteria; the more of these boxes you tick, the more money you earn for your practice. Among them are things like not prescribing expensive antibiotics, or not prescribing too many antibiotics, or keeping within your indicative budget, or not going more than 5% above it. Another revolves around the percentage of generic drugs you prescribe, as opposed to branded ones. When a drug is first released, it is patented. Once the patent runs out, anyone can manufacture it – these 'generics' are cheaper than the original branded drug but generally have exactly the same properties.

As I say, you can't spend your 'budget' and run out of money, but if you bust it you'll end up getting a visit from a Prescribing Advisor from the PCT asking why your prescribing costs were so high and refusing to pay your PIS money. (Unless, of course, you can justify your prescribing. Some years are busier than others.) None of this involves the really expensive blockbuster treatments, like the breast cancer superdrug Herceptin – if someone on your list needs something of this order, you write to the PCT and they will deal with it as an exceptional case.

NHS IT EXPERT — MORON OR OXYMORON? DISCUSS

WITHIN A WEEK or so, the PC doctors had finally fixed the computers and we returned to state normal, where no-one knows what his pills cost.

Next week, something else will go wrong, of course.

I can't for the life of me understand why those in authority place so much faith in computers. This question occurred to me one morning as I attempted, with gritted teeth, to type in a prescription for Mr Snagsby, one of our frequent fliers.

The latest 'helpful update' to the IT systems in our surgery is a program which interrupts me as I'm writing prescriptions for Drug X to inform me that a different drug, Drug Y, would work out 94p per month cheaper.

Because it is a computer system commissioned, designed and implemented by imbeciles, it does not take into account the fact that I know full well that Drug Y is cheaper, but that I have already tried that drug on the patient without success, or have discovered that the patient is dangerously allergic to it, or that I've thought about it but have considered it unsuitable in my professional, that is to say medical, opinion.

Unless I push three different buttons to confirm my original choice, the patient gets switched by a process called ValuScrip to the cheaper version, which is annoying enough.

Worse, though, the PCT are monitoring how many of ValuScrip's recommendations I act on (almost none, as it happens) and they reserve the right to penalise my drug budget by withholding PIS payments if I don't accept a certain proportion of them.

Musing on the difference between a Secretary of State for Health and a GP's computer – chiefly, that you ought only need to punch the information into a Secretary of State once – I eventually achieved the desired result and sent Mr Snagsby on his way with a chit for drugs that may be slightly more expensive than the bean counters would ideally like, but will at least work and have the added benefit of being unlikely to kill him via anaphylactic shock.

It's all of a piece with the 'Connecting for Health' NHS computer system, the black hole that will have swallowed up around £7 billion of our hard-earned tax by the end of 2010. Doctors have been banging on for years about the inadequacies of this programme, with its twilight language of 'Clinical Dashboards Toolkits', 'NHS Interoperability Toolkits' and 'Enterprise-wide Arrangements'.

One aspect of the software is supposed to speed up the process of booking an appointment for a patient to see a consultant. This particular facility is so awful that most GPs refuse to use it, even though patients referred with an old-fashioned letter are theoretically forced to wait longer for their first appointment at the hospital.

The white-coat-and-bow-tie merchants are just as cross about this as GPs, ploughing through clinics full of bunions while little old ladies with painfully crunchy hips are bounced back down the waiting list because their GP sent them along with a handwritten note.

Then there is the issue of security. I've had many patients ask dubiously whether their health records are safe once they are loaded on to the centralised 'NHS spine'. My response: I very much doubt it. The IT nerds insist that electronic records will be more secure than paper-based notes. I look at the almost weekly incidents of thousands of computerised records being left in pubs, emailed to the wrong place or outsourced to India, and then point out that my filing cabinets are locked and I know who has the keys.

The geeks are trying to persuade us that their new systems will improve communication between GPs and hospitals. This is rubbish. My local pathology laboratory installed the latest hideously expensive software a while ago, and the system crashed before the engineer had left the building. For several days, thousands of results had to be faxed or couriered to surgeries while some intensive head-scratching, chocolate-digestive munching and rebooting went on at the lab. When the computer lurched back into action, it sent *seven* copies of *every* test result in its memory into GPs' inboxes, including tests that had been requested by, and should have been reported to, hospital doctors. Then everything crashed again.

The letter of apology that followed was addressed to 67 local GP practices. That's 200 doctors, give or take, who had been repeatedly switching their PCs on and off again after phoning Tech Support.

Still, the technophiles won't give up. Another pilot project allowed patients to see their records and download their test results via the internet. Brilliant – if the scheme is ever rolled out across the country, my patients will be able to discover that they have an inoperable brain tumour from the comfort of their own home. At least that will save me the trouble of my breaking it gently to them.

Why wait? Show up at the surgery with some ID and a few quid and the Data Protection Act ensures that you'll get a printout of your entire computer record: every diagnosis, every prescription, every blood-pressure reading, to do with as you please.

I wonder what you'll make of this:

'TATT 2/52 FH ↓T4 O/E NAD TFT+FBC 2CMA'

Try, 'Tired all The Time, for two weeks, has a Family History of Hypothyroidism, On Examination Nothing Abnormal was Detected, lab rats asked to do some Thyroid Function Tests and a Full Blood Count simply To Cover My Arse.'

MEET REBECCA BAGNET (OR HER DAD, ANYWAY)

AFTER A NOURISHING breakfast of paracetamol on toast and a slug of pholcodine linctus BP, I dragged myself into the surgery today.

You might think that doctors would be good at judging when we're fit for work, considering that a large part of our working day is spent assessing our patients' ability to do jobs we know next to nothing about. Ironically, it isn't so. It's a macho thing: 'proper' doctors don't take sick leave.

First out of the morning's traps was Matthew Bagnet, who had blagged my 8am slot for a prescription review. As he came in he was treated to an exhibition of world class expectoration as I tried to get a particularly stubborn gobbet of phlegm to shift from the back of my throat.

'Blimey, you ought to see a doctor yourself,' he said, as he plonked himself down in the patient's chair and rolled his sleeve up for the ritual blood pressure check.

Wordlessly, I reached into my desk drawer and pulled out a sheet of A4 paper bearing the legend 'YOU SHOULD SEE A DOCTOR'. I crossed out the number 23 and wrote in '24'.

'Ah,' he said. 'You've heard that one before, then.'

It was when we wrapped up his BP check and 12,000 mile service that he hit me with his, 'While I'm here, doc.'

But it wasn't about himself, it was about his daughter, Rebecca. I've seen Rebecca grow up from shy toddler, through highly-strung schoolgirl and into troublesome adolescent.

'It's her diabetes,' he said. 'She's just not taking it seriously.'

He wasn't telling me anything I didn't already know. I'd had a succession of letters from the local Diabetic Day Care Centre, ranging from the straightforward, 'We were sorry that Rebecca couldn't make it in for her assessment today,' to the more recent, 'We really wonder whether it's worth sending this girl any further appointments,' after she failed to attend for the fifth or sixth time.

Along with these there were copies of attendance alerts from A&E departments round and about, all following the same pattern: 'Known insulin-dependant diabetic, low blood sugar, treated and streeted. GP to follow up.'

'OK, Matthew,' I said. 'No more Mr Nice Guy.'

I pulled Rebecca's repeat prescription chart up on the screen, selected 'All Items' and hit the delete button. 'I'm not putting my name to any more insulin scripts until I see some blood numbers, a body mass index and a BP reading on Becca's record. Get her over here before her current supply runs out.'

IMAGINEERING SOLUTIONS FOR SHIFTING PARADIGMS

SAMI AND I HAD a meeting with the PCT suits later.

It all started about a year previously, with a squeal and an expletive from my medical secretary Martha Bardell, both of which were audible from the common room. Such displays of exasperation are unusual from the highly professional and controlled super-sec, so I immediately went to investigate.

I found her hunched over in her chair, slowly banging her head against the desk and moaning.

'Everything alright?' I said, casually.

She looked up and almost growled. 'I don't believe it!' she said. 'It's *another* bloody form!'

More swearing. Blimey! This was serious.

She handed it over. It was, indeed, *another* bloody form. This time, for microscopic haematuria – invisible amounts of blood in your urine. The form – which needed completion by the GP to get the patient referred to a urologist – required around 25 separate pieces of information. Name of patient, obviously. Any abnormal findings on examination, also obviously. But, rather less obviously, questions like, 'Any recent travel?' – perhaps because (and I confess I'm guessing here) obscure tropical diseases can sometimes cause microscopic haematuria.

Anyway. Big deal, you might think. It's just a form. Bite the bullet, fill it in, move on. Fair enough. But then, there's a form for chest pain. And one for indigestion. And another for rectal bleeding. And yet another for headache. And for heavy periods, and infertility, and breathlessness, and memory loss… In fact, no matter what your symptom is, there's a form for it (admittedly, I haven't yet tested this out for the most obscure symptom I can think of, pilimiction – the passage of hairs in your urinary stream – but I have a feeling I wouldn't be disappointed).

There are lots of symptoms, so that's lots of forms. And they need keeping track of, filing and updating, and, of course, the hospital keeps producing new ones and updates on old ones every five minutes. This upsets Martha.

Each form is completely different, each needs tracking down and each needs laborious completion with information that either seems irrelevant or which the hospital doctor is going to get from the patient anyway. And this upsets all of us, because it's a pointless waste of time, effort and, in these recessionary times, money.

Over the following few days, phrases like 'bureaucratic nightmare' and 'unbelievable levels of bullshit' were bandied about, increasingly loudly and vehemently, until, at the next practice meeting, we decided that enough was enough. We would make a stand and stop using those sodding forms. Instead, we reverted to what we'd always done: writing a sensible, courteous referral letter, providing all the information relevant to the particular case but none of the nonsensical frippery.

Brilliant.

Except that, on day three of our brave, form-free world, the first referral bounced back. The next day, a couple were returned. The next, a handful. And then it became apparent that all of our referrals were boomeranging back to us.

Why? To quote the message sent to a molar-grinding Martha, 'These referrals have been refused because your doctors have not used the correct forms.'

This was sorted out by a few choice words directed to some jobsworth on the end of the phone.

'We have a contractual obligation to refer patients to hospital as appropriate,' our Senior Partner told the jobsworth, 'but we are under no obligation whatsoever to use any particular form, any more than we are to fill it in in illuminated script. Which means that, should any patient suffer harm because of your refusal of our referral, medicolegal liability will be held by you.'

This solved the problem. But we'd created such a stir with our policy of non co-operation that the PCT suits weren't happy, which is why Sami and I found ourselves sitting opposite a couple of them this morning.

The meeting went well. Sami explained our position from the outset. He's good at this type of thing: he hates management jargon, but he has a weird talent for it, too.

'The thing is,' he said, 'we don't want our stance to get in the way of a seamless patient journey.'

The suits looked impressed.

'Nor do we want it to reflect badly on our aspiration to Total Quality Management. We'd hate to see a dip in the dials on our Clinical Dashboard.'

The suits glanced approvingly at each other.

'So we've had an idea shower. And, going forward – bear with me – we've come up with a paradigm shift. We'd like to give you the heads up, run it up the flagpole *et cetera*.'

He pulled a piece of paper from his pocket. The suits were obviously intrigued, leaning forward slightly, waiting expectantly for Sami to unveil our masterpiece.

'Clearly,' he continued, 'the status quo isn't a strategic fit for World Class Referring. So we've imagineered a solution.'

Bugger me, he's good. He unfolded the paper.

'We're calling it a "Universal Referral Form", or URF. It's a one-size-fits-all solution. We've cascaded it to local practices and they've all confirmed they think the idea is…'

For the first time, he faltered, searching for the right buzzword. I took this as my cue to chip in.

'They think it's empowering,' I said.

'Exactly!' said Sami. 'They think it's empowering.'

The suits could barely contain their excitement.

'We think we can work synergistically with you to facilitate this across all practices,' said Sami, recovering his poise and handing over our meisterwork. 'It's kind of a win-win-win. You, us and the patients.'

The suits looked blank. As did the piece of paper they were holding.

'This is a piece of headed notepaper?' said Suit one, slowly.

'With nothing on it?' said Suit two.

'That's right,' beamed Sami. 'On which we write a referral letter. A Universal Referral Form, like I said. We'd like to enter it for the Strategic Health Authority's annual awards. The "Innovation" section. If you could just sign our entry here?'

'Are you sure you've used the right entry form, Sami?' I said.

CHARLIE DARNAY AND ME

TWO MONTHS AGO, Charlie Darnay, a bright bloke in his mid 20s who was studying hard for a challenging IT qualification, came to see me. He complained of a variety of things – *inter alia*, that he couldn't sleep, he had aches and pains in his joints, a persistent sore throat, problems concentrating, short-term memory lapses and occasional dizziness and nausea. If he did any exercise, such as the weekly game of squash that he used to enjoy, things got worse rather than better. His performance at college was suffering and he was worried sick that he'd fail his next set of exams.

I ran some blood tests to check for various possibilities, such as anaemia, diabetes and thyroid trouble, and they all came up blank.

I had him in again to decide where to go next.

'The results were all inconclusive,' I said. 'We can rule out anything really serious, I think, but…'

'Could it be ME, doctor?' he said. 'My girlfriend was reading about it in one of her magazines and it sounds like what I've got.'

'Hmmm,' I said. 'Well, your symptoms certainly fit the diagnostic criteria.'

ME – short for myalgic encephalomyelitis, and also known as chronic fatigue syndrome (CFS) – is a controversial condition, with attitudes ranging from those who doubt its very existence to those for whom it seems to be their *raison d'être*. Things get surprisingly heated in both camps, especially considering that we're dealing with people who say they're suffering from very low levels of energy. Whatever. There's a bloke in the Rheumatology Department at the local hospital – Dr Snitchey – for whom it's a special interest. Not long back, I attended a lecture he gave about the issue and he seemed a good sort; the obvious thing to do was to get Charlie and Dr Snitchey together.

You may have heard of the new NHS system called Choose and Book which – in theory – entitles patients to choose when and where they go for treatment. The thing is, it's a pretty complicated and exhausting process, and since Charlie was *already* exhausted he asked me to sort it out for him.

This is where it gets irritating.

'So, can you arrange for me to see this Dr Snitchey, then?' said Charlie.

'I'd like to send you to see him,' I said, 'but I… er… can't.'

'You can't?' said Charlie. 'But I thought you said he was an expert in the field?'

'He is,' I said. 'Not that long ago – I mean, only five or ten years back – it would all have been very straightforward. I would have written a letter directly to Dr Snitchey via his secretary, and you would have toddled off to see him in his clinic. Job done. Unfortunately, we're not allowed to book like this any more.'

'You're not?'

'No.'

'So what do you do?'

'These days, I have to write a general referral letter to the hospital. All I can really do is address it to Dr Snitchey, with strict instructions that only he or his secretary opens it, making it plain that you need to see him, and hope for the best.'

'Well, surely if it's addressed to him he'll open it and they'll just book me in with him?' said Charlie.

'I wish it were that simple,' I said, 'but, in my experience, what will probably happen is that the letter will find its way to the Referral Management Centre.'

'What's that?'

'It's a room somewhere with a lot of computer screens and telephones where they collect all the hospital referrals sent up by GPs and decide who the patients get to see.'

'Right,' said Charlie, looking puzzled. 'So surely *they'll* send me on to Dr Snitchey then?'

'Hmmm,' I said. 'You'd like to think so, wouldn't you? Unfortunately, they don't take much notice of what we write in our letters. They tend to make up their own minds as to what treatment you need.'

'But at least they're doctors, right? The people in this Referral Management Centre?'

'Er, no. They're just bodies sat in front of computers, ticking boxes and pushing paper. The chances are they will see that the letter has been addressed to a consultant in the rheumatology department, so you'll end up being sent to a consultant in that department, but not necessarily Dr Snitchey.'

Which is exactly what happened.

Charlie entered the twilight world of the Referral Management Centre, they ignored my request and arranged instead for him to see Dr Snitchey's colleague, Dr Craggs. Craggs is perfectly capable when it comes to arthritis and systemic lupus erythematosus, but has no interest or expertise whatsoever in chronic fatigue syndrome.

This morning I received notice from the hospital telling me that Dr Craggs had examined Charlie and that he felt, on reflection, that he would have been better off seeing his recently-appointed colleague Dr Snitchey who works just down the corridor. Snitchey has special expertise in the management of these cases, don'tcha know?

Yes, I do – but a fat lot of good it did me or my patient.

REFERRAL MANAGEMENT CENTRES

IF THIS REFERRAL Management Centre business all sounds confusing, that's because (like almost everything else in the NHS) it is. One of the problems in writing about this stuff is that the systems keep changing. Also, different systems operate in different areas of the country. (OK, that's two problems).

The RMCs are run by PCTs and are supposed to lead to a more streamlined service, but unfortunately when you insert a layer of non-medical pen-pushers into the process and allow them to interpret GP referrals as they see fit, the result is anything but. My patients are often sent to the wrong specialists, which obviously annoys everyone – me, the patients and the specialists. (Martha, my medical secretary, is forever dealing with complaints from hospital consultants that the wrong type of problem is ending up in the wrong type of clinic).

It can be relatively minor – Charlie won't be dying of tiredness – but it can be very serious. For instance, a friend of mine referred a 38-year-old man with protein and microscopic haematuria in his urine. As any medical fule kno, this man needs to see a renal physician, since this is likely to be an inherent renal problem – unlike where the problem is of microscopic blood in the urine alone, in which case he needs to see a urologist for a standard package of tests (ultrasound of the renal tract, cystoscopy to peer into his bladder) to exclude stones and tumours etc. My friend referred the patient (correctly) with the blood + protein scenario to renal; RMC sees 'blood in urine', so diverts the patient to urology. The patient was scheduled for cystoscopy – an invasive procedure he *didn't* need which had the added effect of delaying the tests he *did* need. It's bonkers and dangerous.

For more on Referral Management Centres, see the NHS Institute for Innovation and Improvement website (and have a glass of whisky and a service revolver handy).

CHARLIE DARNAY, ME AND CHOOSE AND BOOK

WHAT IF CHARLIE hadn't been quite as tired as he was, and had exercised his legal right to use the aforementioned 'Choose and Book' to arrange the time and place of his treatment?

The government's 'Choice Agenda' boast is that 'service users' like Charlie can make these decisions for themselves if they want to, as long as the place they choose meets NHS standards and costs. They can make this choice based on a large number of criteria, from the serious (clinical performance or waiting time) to the relatively trivial (parking facilities).

This might sound like a great idea – it's so much better than someone like me dictating to Charlie where he's going, surely? And not only will he get a say in his care, but it will also improve that care: the modern NHS is funded under a system called 'Payment by Results', under which the money is supposed to follow the patient. Patient choice will provide hospitals with an incentive to improve the quality of their services to attract more patients. Or so the theory says.

In reality, it isn't that simple.

How wide *is* Charlie's choice?

The Choose and Book website says: 'Choose and Book is a service that lets you choose... any hospital in England funded by the NHS. You can choose the date and time of your appointment.'

Pretty unequivocal. But later, it admits that it only promises that 'in most cases' he can choose the date and time of his appointment. There's a good chance that actually the exact time and date he wants won't be available. Is this a minor quibble, or a major get-out? You decide.

Secondly, sure, he can choose his hospital by going onto the NHS Choices website. In the Brave New World of the joined-up NHS, the government thinks this is easy, but then the Secretary of State for Health won't have to use the system. Here's the reality.

Charlie goes online and clears the first hurdle – the web browser he uses actually allows him to view the site. You'd think this would be a given, but the 'Frequently Asked Questions' for Choose and Book somehow manage to say both of the following:

> **Why was I told my browser was not compatible when I tried to log into the Choose and Book service?**
>
> *Some browsers didn't used to work* (sic) *with the Choose and Book service, but we have now made sure that all browsers will work with the service.*

and

> **Why doesn't Choose and Book work with my web browser?**
>
> *The Choose and Book patient application is compatible with all versions of Internet Explorer and with the latest version of Firefox. Whilst we*

> *accept that this does not make the site accessible*
> *to everybody at this time, we are working hard to*
> *ensure 100% accessibility as soon as possible.*

Go figure.

So Charlie hits the button marked 'Find and choose services – Hospitals' and types in his home address.

Whooooah! Up comes the following boast: 'We found 299 hospitals within 50 miles of your address.'

Well, this is all supposed to be about choice, and to get the best you may have to travel. So if he really wants to, Charlie can now start ploughing through this enormous list to find the hospital rated highest for the treatment he needs.

This is by no means a simple task, as the site repeatedly admits: *'We are aware of the treatment names on this page can be confusing.'* (sic)

He chooses a hospital at random and finds himself enmeshed in a complex maze of Care Quality Commission jargon, downloadable .pdf files and click-throughs:

- Full details about which standards this organisation met in 2008/2009
- Read Clareshire NHS Trust's declaration and the information we used to check it
- General statement by Clareshire NHS Trust
- Statement by the patient and public involvement forum
- Statement by overview and scrutiny committee
- Statement by the strategic health authority
- Trust's response to the hygiene code
- Signatories
- Additional information

- More about how we assess whether organisations are meeting core standards
- See how Clareshire NHS Trust results compare with other healthcare organisations in England.

Remember, these are just a small part of the data on one hospital.

It's a good job Charlie's IT-savvy, because if you're not, trust me, you could spend days wandering around here. As it is, realistically, it could take him hours. And hours.

He clicks back out to the main directory. In some cases, it simply isn't clear whether the hospitals listed do or do not offer the relevant service (*'We currently have no information on patient services for this hospital'*); where they do, much of the information as to the quality of the service delivered is presented in confusing, multicoloured bar charts, with multiple click-throughs to detailed pages discussing whether the hospital is meeting things called 'core standards', 'existing commitments' and 'national priorities' which, I predict, mean very little to you. Care Quality Commission ratings from 'excellent' through 'good' and 'fair' to 'weak' litter his screen. Details as to car parking and whether the wards have pay TVs are sometimes easier to find than more important issues like the mortality rate or prevailing incidence of MRSA or C. diff (*'Data not available'*).

Charlie clicks back out to the original screen. Does he really want to spend the rest of the weekend selecting one of 299 hospitals to use? Does he want to travel 25 miles for treatment? Unlike many of my patients, he does have a car. But then, like a lot of people who need to go to hospital, he's also knackered. He narrows the search down to a more manageable 10 miles from his home address.

This produces a list of five hospitals. A bit more like it.

However, of these, only one actually offers the services he requires – and, unsurprisingly, it's the hospital I would have directed him to anyway.

So much for 'choice'.

Using his 'unique NHS reference number' and a password, he can now book his appointment online or by telephone to a call centre halfway across the country.

Well, you might say – apart from the fact that the Choose and Book USP is a bit misleading (Charlie *might* not get the time he wants, and he's basically chosen the nearest hospital to him, as most people do) and apart from the fact that it has taken him a long and frustrating time to get to this point – what's the problem?

The problem is this: while Charlie can choose the time and place of his treatment, what he has given up – without even realising it – is the chance to choose the *specialist*.

OK, a Department of Health spokesperson will be quick to point out here that Charlie never *literally* had a choice of specialist in the past, either. Strictly speaking, this would be true. But *I* did, and I, as his advocate, would make the best choice I possibly could for him, based on my knowledge of who's who, who's interested in what and which consultant answers to 'Two Brains' rather than 'Dumbo'.

Remember, I know our friend Snitchey and his interest in CFS/ ME, and I'd have sent him direct to Snitchey.

But all Charlie can do is book to see *someone* in the rheumatology department, where there are a bunch of other doctors, who are all perfectly capable when it comes to crunchy joints and brittle bones, but none of whom share this interest in patients with chronic fatigue.

Eventually, of course, one of them will direct him to Dr Snitchey, but only after months of wasted time.

SHOULDERING THE BURDEN

FUNNILY ENOUGH, the very next patient I had in had experienced similar problems.

He was Mr Marley, he was favouring his right shoulder, and he wasn't very bloody happy.

'I'm on the mend, doctor,' he said. '*Finally*. But I'm not very bloody happy.'

I said I didn't blame him, and that neither was I.

Mr Marley first came to see me six months ago. He's a keen veteran rugby player, and he'd knackered the shoulder while tackling a 20-stone behemoth on the hoof.

'I'm way too old for this game, doc,' he'd said, ruefully. 'I reckon that's my last match for the Old Stupidians.'

I examined him. It looked like a pretty straightforward shoulder impingement – this is where the tendons around the shoulder blade and the humerus, or upper arm, are damaged and inflamed. It's painful and quite debilitating, and, given that Mr Marley's job as a courier involved driving, lifting and carrying, it was quite a problem for him.

We put him in a sling, injected the inflamed area with cortisone and dosed him up with anti-inflammatories. Once the initial problem had started to subside, I sent him for some physiotherapy.

Usually, all of this does the trick but in this case it didn't. He got back some mobility, and could just about function in his day-to-day life, but he couldn't work properly and was still in quite a lot of pain. I saw him again a month or so after the injury, re-examined him and decided that he needed a subacromial decompression.

'Basically, that's an operation to clear out the crap which has built up in the joint and is preventing it from healing properly,' I said.

'I don't fancy going under the knife,' he said.

'I don't blame you,' I said. 'Hospitals are dangerous. If the sleep-deprived junior doctor don't get you, MRSA will.'

I grinned, but it was only partially a joke. A while ago, a consultant chest physician called Professor Sherwood Burge was all over the papers when he admitted that his hospital was 'not a terribly safe place to be'. Like this was news! In common with a lot of GPs, I do my best to keep my patients away from hospitals. All blood samples for routine tests are done at my surgery rather than at the pathology lab, and I send them over there for X-rays and scans only when there's a real chance that the results might influence their treatment (more importantly, this helps to keep the place freed up for those who really need it). I go to great lengths to avoid showing my own face there, too.

'Having said that,' I went on, 'it's a fairly routine procedure – a keyhole thing. It doesn't take too long, and you'll be up and out of hospital in no time.'

'Well,' he said. 'Anything to get this sorted, I suppose.'

This is when the problems really started.

In the old days, I'd have referred Mr Marley direct to my mate in orthopaedics who happens to have a special interest in shoulder problems, and Mr Marley would have been in the diary for the following Tuesday. (This would happen on the basis that I am a fairly good GP and I didn't mess them around; bad GPs who consistently referred rubbish might tend to find their referrals delayed for a bit.)

To refer someone nowadays, I have to fill in a stack of paperwork and fight my way through a dozen secretaries, managers and commissars. I duly did all of this, specifying quite clearly that Mr Marley needed this operation. I've been a general practitioner for 20 years, I've seen a lot of knackered shoulders and I don't refer people for surgery willy-nilly. If I say he needs an op, he needs an op. You might assume, naively, that I was referring him to an orthopaedic surgeon for that op. Mr Marley certainly did.

The bureaucrats thought otherwise. Instead, they diverted Mr Marley away to the 'Consultant Upper Limb Nurse Practitioner' – a stupid, aggrandised title which basically means 'jumped-up physio'.

The CULNP didn't 'fess up to this when he saw Mr Marley, of course, and instead relied heavily on the word 'Consultant' in his job title, so the patient *thought* he was seeing a proper specialist, as per my directions. The CULNP spent the next two months fannying around doing more and more physio until he finally began to suspect what I already knew and had already requested: that Mr Marley needed a subacromial decompression. Brilliant.

I only found this out when the CULNP wrote to me in a slightly high-handed way telling me to arrange a scan. Then I got a further letter which had me bouncing off the walls in rage.

Dear Dr Copperfield, it said. *The MRI scan has revealed that Mr Marley requires a surgical decompression. Would you please refer him for this procedure.*

Aaaarrrrggghh! I already effing have – last autumn.

On Monday, six months, two weeks and three days after wandering off the rugby pitch in a daze, Mr Marley finally had the op he needed.

When he came in to see me yesterday he wanted some co-codamol painkillers.

'Bloody hell, doctor,' he said. 'I've been off work for ages. I'm lucky I ain't been fired. What the hell was that all about?'

That's a very good question.

WHAT *WAS* IT ALL ABOUT?

WHAT IT WAS all about was waiting lists and money.

The hospitals will say that it isn't, and that it's all down to GPs for sending them crap referrals which could have been dealt with without surgery. Sure, there are some of those. But the fact is most of us know what we're doing and we don't ask them to cut our patients open unless they really need it.

Politically, the Health Minister wants to be able to stand up in Parliament – or put out a press release – saying that he will ensure that you will see a consultant inside 18 weeks.

The hospitals and Trusts need to hit that target, because there are all sorts of bonuses and promotions tied up with doing so, and lots of bad headlines and sackings (well, bad headlines) if they don't.

The problem is, consultant surgeons cost lots of money and in the real world there aren't enough of them to cover everything.

We ought to be able to explain this to people. 'I'm really sorry, I know you're supposed to see Mr Mulberry-Hawk within 18 weeks, but there's been a rash of broken wrists thanks to the cold winter and the system's creaking a bit… can you wait a bit longer?'

But for some reason we don't, so when Mr Marley arrives at the hospital, they shunt him off to the 'Consultant Upper Limb Nurse Practitioner' and tick a box on the computer saying that he was seen within the 18 week limit.

The treatment he needs – and which we've always known he needs – actually takes forever, and he may lose his job while waiting for it, but at least the Health Minister can't be embarrassed in the press.

This isn't the only way they game* the system. You can't have surgery if your blood pressure's high, so when you attend for your pre-operative assessment clinic, don't be surprised if the nurse starts telling you all about the possible complications of your aortic aneurysm – like death, to name but one. It's only fair, after all, that you are properly informed, and if the side effect of that is that it terrifies you so much that your BP shoots up to two points over normal for the first time in your life, so you can't have the op because the protocol says you can't, and the waiting list clock starts all over again, tough. Sorry, you'll just have to go back to your GP and get him to re-refer you when your blood pressure's OK. And by the way, here's a letter to your GP telling him he's pretty useless for referring you with high blood pressure in the first place.

It was fine until you walked up behind him and went BOO! you bastard.

*OK, it may not actually be gaming – though part of me thinks it just might be – but it is bloody stupid, thoughtless, protocol-driven medicine which drives me and the punters mad.

KAFKAESQUE

I'M REALLY NOT saying everything was better years ago and that it's all rubbish now, because it wasn't and it isn't, but try this one on for size.

I had a patient recently who I was pretty sure had developed multiple sclerosis. I wanted her seen urgently for an MRI scan and a lumbar puncture to test her cerebrospinal fluid for certain MS markers.

The hospital came back to me with an appointment: 11.30am on May 15. Given that this was, at that point, more than four months away, I felt they were stretching the definition of 'urgent' somewhat.

I called the relevant department and spoke to a secretary there.

'Hello, it's Dr Copperfield from Bleak House,' I said. 'I asked for my patient Mrs Dedlock to be seen urgently for an MRI and some tests. You've come back with 11.30am on May 15. Can you please explain to me how that fits the definition of "urgent"?'

'Well, we are very busy, doctor,' she said.

'And Mrs Dedlock is very poorly,' I said. 'Potentially very poorly indeed. So I need her seeing pronto. Can you have a look in your diary and find me something quicker, please?'

There was a sigh and the sound of fingers clicking on a keyboard. In the background, I could hear dozens of other office-dwellers merrily gossiping with each other. The secretary came back to me.

'As I say, doctor, we really are very busy. But I have managed to find you an earlier appointment for the patient.'

There was a pause. I think she was expecting me to prostrate myself telephonically before her and sob in gratitude.

'Yes?' I said. 'What is it?'

'It's 11am on May 15,' she said.

'What?'

'It's 11am, May 15.'

'Are you winding me up?'

'Er, no. Why?'

'I ring you with a very sick patient, a mother of three who I am pretty sure is about to be told she has multiple sclerosis. I point out that the appointment you have given her is more than four months in the future and ask for her to be seen sooner than that. And you give me an appointment half an hour earlier? Half a bloody hour?'

'Well... '

'I'm ringing you in premium appointment time, here,' I said, frothing slightly at the mouth. 'I have patients waiting outside the door, and I'm on to you having a conversation like this? Are you mad?'

We got Mrs Dedlock seen much quicker, but how much time and angst does this sort of thing take up?

And if you think that's an isolated case, think again. I could give you dozens of similar examples.

Not long after that debacle, I was consulted by Mr Tulkinghorn, a man in his 40s, who was having chest pain. I referred him to hospital, the problem settled down and they allowed him to go home. I then got an email asking me to arrange for Mr Tulkinghorn to have a stress test on his heart, followed by an appointment with the consultant cardiologist so that the results could be evaluated. (Quite why the hospital cannot arrange this test and the appointment themselves I'm not sure – they used to, but nowadays it all comes back to us. Actually, scratch that: I *am* sure. In our pointlessly complex funding system, if it's not arranged by the GP, the hospital doesn't get funded for it, or not funded so much, or something like that, so everything they would have previously sorted themselves – obviously quicker and more sensible – gets bounced back to us.)

With horrible inevitability, Mr Tulkinghorn was given his cardiology appointment *before* the stress test. I called the hospital to try to sort it out. They cancelled the appointment with the consultant, because there was no point in him being seen until he'd had the stress test. The patient then got a letter saying: 'You did not attend for your appointment. You must go back to your GP to be re-referred.'

By now, it was quite possible I'd be needing a cardiology appointment of my own: God knows what this mad, circular, bureaucratic nonsense does to the poor patients.

Perhaps the best example of this insanity involved a 70-year-old patient with an iffy heart, arterial disease all over the place and one leg amputated as a result of his vascular problems. He was due to see the heart specialist when his health took a nosedive from 'seriously ill' to 'just about dead' and he was rushed in to have the other leg chopped off. As a result of this, he was going to miss his cardiology appointment. His wife rang Outpatients to apologise and ask if they could rearrange it. The response she received was: *This is not sufficient excuse for missing his appointment. His GP must book another one.*

I know this sounds so surreal that Salvador Dali would have dismissed it as implausible, but I swear I'm not making it up.

I was so angry that I actually sent a letter to the powers-that-be at the hospital.

> *Dear X, I said. I write with regard to my patient, Mr Young, and your recent conversation with his wife. Just for future reference, can you please tell me what criteria you think you might accept as 'sufficient' for missing an appointment? Because it seems to me that being rushed in to have your only remaining fucking leg cut off ought to score pretty high?*

After writing it, I started to worry that I was being too aggressive – a clear sign that I am losing it. I showed it to Sami Patel. 'I'd take out the "fucking",' he said. 'Otherwise, spot on.'

I'LL TELL YOU WHY
I DON'T LIKE MONDAYS

TODAY WAS THE second Monday of the month, and that means it was our monthly partnership meeting.

O joy of joys.

These meetings involve the four partners (the Senior Partner, myself, Sami and Amy Daniels, struggling in from maternity leave) and the practice manager SS-Obersturmbannführer Jane Carstone. We kick off at around 8pm, we talk about the future of the practice and its staff, and we grind on until we are all either dead or prepared to concede anything to anyone, usually just in time for last orders.

First item on the agenda was a complaint to Jane that I had spoken too sharply to one of the receptionists, Gordon.

'Mrs Peggotty says you were rude to Gordon,' she said. 'Apparently, you said to him, and I quote: "Why don't you just piss off, you are a bloody moron at times".'

'Well, to be honest I wouldn't be distraught if he did leave,' I said. 'He's hopeless. He loses paperwork, he irritates the sane patients and encourages the nutters and he consistently puts phone calls through to surgery when he knows he shouldn't. All that said, I didn't tell him to piss off. I may have been looking in his general direction, but I was talking to Dr Patel at the time. As he will confirm.'

Sami nodded. 'It's true,' he said.

'Two things,' said Jane, coolly. 'Number one: I know Gordon has some performance issues, but if you have any problem with him there are procedures which must be followed...'

'Und orders vhich *vill* be obeyed,' said Sami Patel.

'...and number two: do you really think that two partners should be talking to each other like that in front of the staff? And potentially patients?'

'Fair point,' I said. 'But he *is* a moron.'

'Fair point,' nodded Sami.

'Next,' said Jane. 'Just to note that the new registrar, Lucie Manette, joins in a fortnight.' About one quarter of GP practices are approved for training, and ours is one of them. Trainee GPs in their final year are called registrars; most stay with you for a year, heavily supervised, with lots of tutorials and paperwork. A good one means you have, in effect, an extra partner for a year. A bad one means you have a nightmare. 'She'll initially work out of Amy's room while she's off on maternity, if that's OK with you?'

'Fine,' said Amy.

'Is she the tall blonde who was here last week?' said Sami. 'She looks as though she has bags of potential.'

'She is tall and she is blonde, Dr Patel,' said Jane. 'Are you insinuating something?'

Sami just grinned.

'Next,' said Jane. 'The new Darzi Polyclinic opens in Skimpole Street this spring. We still have to decide what to do about that.'

These Darzi's Khazis were proposed by the former Health Minister Ara Darzi a while back. The basic idea is that you have everything – from primary care to minor surgery to dentistry to counselling – under one roof. We GPs don't think they can do what we do as well as we do it, or what hospitals, dentists and head doctors do as well as *they* do it, and instead are a bit of a mess. There are arguments the other way, too, although most pander to the time-pressured worried well, rather than the elderly or chronically sick who have health 'needs' rather than 'wants'. But one thing is certain, they do threaten the future of general practice, and are radically changing the way we work. For starters, they're open from 8am until 8pm, seven days a week. Another issue is that you don't *have* to register with them to be seen – you just walk in off the street. It's not hard to see how patients might decide not to register with us, and with so much of a practice's income linked to the size of its patient list, there are obvious risks here, both for us GPs and for patients: namely, the loss of fluffy things like continuity and personalised care, with the caring, friendly visage of the family doctor being replaced by some faceless unknown whose main concern is finishing his shift on time.

'As I see it,' said Sami, 'we either open longer and all work longer hours, or we lose patients. And we don't want to lose patients, do we?'

'We could take on another salaried partner,' said the Senior Partner.

Salaried GPs earn around £60k or £70k a year and are the Ronnie Woods of medicine: they turn up, play guitar (or dish out scripts) and go home. They don't attend partnership meetings, don't have a say in how the place is run and generally act as a bum on a seat during the grotty late night and weekend shifts. Sometimes, they are docs who have no interest in a partnership for personal reasons – as with our current salaried employee, Dr Emma. (In her case, it's because committing to the practice would mean getting involved in the admin and the non-clinical stuff which sends us bonkers, while interfering in her regular trips overseas to save whales, bond with the Inuit and harvest free trade knitwear in the favelas of São Paulo.) In other instances, they'd love a partnership but the partners won't give them one because they turn out to be rubbish, or mad, or weird, or all three.

'It might sound radical,' I said, 'but, actually, would it be such a nightmare to lose a few patients? Do we really want to hang on to the people who want to be seen at 8.30pm for a sore throat? Let them go down the Darzi, I say – 10% of our patients cause 90% of our workload, so if we lost the *right* 10% we'd be quids in, relatively-speaking. We could get rid of Dr Emma, never mind take on a new bod.'

'You really are all heart, Tony,' said Amy.

'We're not getting rid of Emma,' said Sami. 'What are you on about?'

'We certainly don't want to lose patients,' said the Senior Partner. 'Thin end of the wedge, that sort of thing.'

'So are you going to up your hours? Or should we look at another salaried doctor?' said Jane Carstone.

'If we really don't want to shed a few punters then maybe we should look at the salaried option to supply some extra hours,' I said.

'The only thing is, if we take someone else on... what if we rearrange all the rotas and then they don't like it, or they don't fit in?' said Amy. 'What with me being off at the moment...'

'If they don't fit in, we'll get another,' I said. 'There's an endless supply of them.'

'Why don't you knock up a bit of a plan and we'll vote on it at the next meeting, Jane?' said the Senior Partner, to general nods of agreement.

'Next,' said Jane. 'Just to note that the insurance premiums are due for payment and are going up again.'

There were groans around the table. Not that long ago, our profession was up in arms when annual premiums broke through the £1,000 mark. Now, thanks to ambulance-chasing lawyers, I pay £5,000 a year so that my arse is covered when I kill you because I supposedly didn't tell you not to wash your warfarin down with a couple of bottles of wine.

'A chap I know has just cut his week down to three days,' said the Senior Partner. 'His insurance premiums are down by a thousand pounds. He's earning less, but with the new top rate tax thingy...'

'He sounds like a very socially responsible bloke, your mate,' said Sami.

'You may very well be the first Hero of the Revolution to drive a Porsche Boxter,' I said.

The agenda moved on to our locum, Gavin. He's been with us ever since Amy decided having another child was a sensible option. Although locums can earn very good money – £90 an hour, or around

£175k a year, *pro rata* – he's permanently broke, due to several failed marriages and a large number of squealing progeny.

'Gavin's been offered a partnership in Bristol,' said Jane. 'It's near his kids by his second wife…'

'Third,' said Sami.

'It's near his kids by his third wife, so he's accepted. He joins in three months, so there's plenty of time to arrange another for the period before Amy comes back.'

'And by then we'll know what the new registrar's like,' I pointed out. 'If she cuts the mustard, we might not need an extra pair of hands.'

'Tony, I'm surprised to have to remind you that registrars are here to learn, not be exploited,' said Jane. 'Lucie certainly couldn't be expected to do extended hours while the rest of you swan off.'

'True,' agreed Sami. 'Nice idea, though. Be a shame to lose Gavin. I'll miss lending him a tenner for his lunch three times a week.'

The meeting rambled on in this style for the next hour or two, until Jane called for any other business.

Sami stuck a hand up. 'I've got something I want to raise,' he said, looking at me. 'I heard you talking to Nurse Susie the other day, Copperfield.'

'And?' I said.

'And she was moaning about having to tick boxes and fill in forms to chase QOF points, and you said you knew how she felt, it was a pain in the arse.'

QOF points are an expensive new bureaucratic way of paying us to do things we already did. I'll explain them more fully in a moment.

'It *is* a pain in the arse,' I said. 'I do object to having some highly-paid, chairbound biro-jockey hovering over my shoulder checking how many of our bloody diabetics we've tested for sodding micro-albuminuria in the last 15 months. Or worrying about whether we have a written policy for responding to requests for emergency contraception. Or docking us points for forgetting to tick a box which says there's no issue outstanding if a patient is up for a medication review and there's no fucking issue outstanding.'

'Listen, you pillock,' said Sami. 'You can't say stuff like that to the nurses. They *should* be filling out the forms, that's how we make a living! How can we bollock them for not doing it if they hear you moaning about it?'

'Who's behind with his blood tests?' I said. 'Do I need to remind you of Hypothyroidism Indicator 2, "Ongoing Management: The percentage of patients with hypothyroidism with thyroid function tests recorded in the previous 15 months"? You've got stacks of outstanding tests, and that's six QOF points going begging unless you get your act together.'

'They're being sorted,' he said. 'I had a problem with my computer, as you well know.'

'Children, children,' said the Senior Partner. 'Can we agree that QOF points equals profits, and since partners share profits we need to do all we can to ensure we harvest as many QOF points as possible? That means encouraging the staff to stick needles in anything which moves and make a note of so doing, *and* making sure we do the same.'

That's general practice: a constant tension between trying to get on with being a good professional and the distraction of proving that I'm doing so, just so I can pay the mortgage. Something I could have said, at this point. But I didn't. Instead, I suggested we adjourn to the Red Lion.

QOF POINTS

I'M SORRY TO say that this explanation will be very tedious, and will contain lots of typically convoluted and labyrinthine NHS bureaucratese ('...they are derived from the Quality Management Analysis System [QMAS], a national IT system developed by NHS Connecting for Health...'), and that at the end of it all you may be left scratching your head and wondering why they bothered. You're not alone.

The Quality and Outcomes Framework (QOF) is a national system introduced with the General Medical Services (GMS) contract on – fittingly enough – April Fool's Day, 2004.

Under QOF, the idea is that each GP practice is measured in a variety of areas so that patients, PCTs and politicians can judge us against a mythical average standard, instead of trusting us, as professionals, to do a job that few of them actually understand.

These areas are called 'Domains', and there are four of them: the 'Clinical Domain', the 'Organisational Domain', the 'Patient Experience Domain' and the 'Additional Services Domain'. Each 'Domain' is split into 'Areas' (28 in total) which are themselves further sub-divided into 129 'Indicators'.

We get awarded 'QOF points' for ticking the myriad boxes in these Domains, and we get money for each QOF point. There are a total of 1,000 QOF points on offer, and each point is worth £124.60 (adjusted for 'prevalence' and the 'contractor population index', which really are too boring to go into).

As a for instance, the biggest of the 'Areas' in the 'Clinical Domain' is Coronary Heart Disease, which has 10 'Indicators'.

To take one at random, 'CHD 3' is: 'The percentage of patients with coronary heart disease, whose notes record smoking status in the past 15 months, except those who have never smoked where smoking status need be recorded only once.'

If we hit a target of 90% – i.e., 90% of patients have this box ticked in their medical notes – we earn seven QOF points.

To take another, 'BP 3' is: 'The percentage of patients with hypertension [high blood pressure] who smoke, whose notes contain a record that smoking cessation advice has been offered at least once.'

If we hit 90% here, by telling smokers to give up, we earn ten more QOF points.

In a way, it's all rather insulting. The insinuation – perhaps even the accusation – is that we really don't give a stuff about our patients and cannot be trusted to do the best for them, that if you attend my surgery as a 40-a-day man with a dodgy ticker or high blood pressure, without the government sitting on my back and, er, dangling QOF carrots in my face, I won't bother telling you to stop tabbing.

Ah well, you say, you're a big boy, Copperfield – you can live with the odd mild insult here and there from whoever is Health Secretary this week.

That's true, but what do you think the outcome of QOF was?

When the QOF target-setting team asked GPs how much preventive medicine we already practised, we told them and they didn't believe us. They set the average QOF score at 700 out of a possible 1,050 points a year (it was later reduced to the current 1,000), and decreed that any GP scoring more than 700 points would get a proportional pay rise. Most doctors immediately scored over 800 with minimal extra effort, simply by using the first few minutes of each consultation to tick the boxes on their screens which confirmed what they already did: 'Patient has been advised to stop smoking; use condoms; eat fruit; lose weight; exercise more; drink less.'

In fact, across the piece, we managed to earn 90% of the available points, and now we all drive Maseratis.

The Maserati bit is a joke, although we do earn more than they thought we would, but it is true that all that has really happened is I now spend my time filling in forms which an NHS bureaucrat employed in an office somewhere spends time auditing, before another NHS bureaucrat in another office somewhere spends time collating, before another NHS bureaucrat in another office somewhere sends me some money for doing what I already did but perhaps didn't always write down in a prescribed format.

It's always nice earning more, but when you add up the cost of QOF and QMAS and NHS Connecting for Health, I can't help wondering whether it was all either necessary, or good value for taxpayers' money, or made any significant difference to actual patients.

GOING POSTAL

I ARRIVED AT work at 7.15am to see Mrs Peggotty struggling manfully to heft two big black bags into one of the large trolley bins in the car park.

I'd have offered to help, but it was raining cats and dogs and I didn't want to put my back out, so I ducked down below the dashboard – to re-tie my shoelace, you understand, not so that she wouldn't see me – and waited. It took her ages, mostly using the clean-and-jerk technique, but eventually she managed to shoulder them into the bins. I sprang from the Nissan and got to the entrance door just in time to hold it open for her.

'After you, Mrs Peggotty,' I said. 'Terrible weather, isn't it?'

'I saw you in your car there, Dr Copperfield,' she said. 'I was thinking perhaps you'd give me a hand. Those bags were awful heavy, like. All that junk mail.'

'I'm awfully sorry, Mrs Peggotty, but I didn't... my lace... oh, crumbs, is that the time? Surgery starts in... I must...'

Safely ensconced at my desk with a mug of coffee, I found myself confronted by a pile of letters approximately six inches thick. It's like this most mornings, and a week from now plucky old Mrs Peggotty will be back out by the trolley bins, girding her loins for another struggle with 100 kilos of pointless paper.

The first seven or eight envelopes were franked with pharmaceutical company logos, which at least saved me the trouble of opening them. Such letters are always either trying to market a drug I won't use, or inviting me to an educational event (with free meal) to teach me about a drug I don't want to know about, or informing me that either of the aforementioned two drugs have been withdrawn due to unforeseen problems (but that's OK, because I won't have prescribed them anyway).

There was a pile of casualty slips telling me that patient X attended our local A&E with Y and had Z done to him. Obviously, I read these, though they often can leave you more confused than if you hadn't. They're produced on a computer *proforma* and because the diagnosis often isn't clear and the staff are in such a hurry, they often make no sense at all. For example, the first one read:

> Patient attended with: *Head.*
> Diagnosis: *Other.*
> Management: *Returned to GP.*

Er, thanks.

There were one or two letters from the hospital telling me about patients who have had recent clinic appointments or in-patient stays. These are read – or at least scanned (and sometimes laughed at, for similar reasons to the A&E reports).

A quick slurp of now-lukewarm coffee, and I moved on to the requests for reports for life insurance or assurance, allowances, disabled parking stickers, and fitness to appear on television game shows (yes, really).

My eye strayed to the clock on my wall: 7.45am. Fifteen more minutes, and then the first patient of the day would be bashing down my door.

I finished the coffee and returned to the now-smaller pile of mail.

A fat brown envelope ('All our junk is printed on recycled paper originally sourced from environmentally sustainable forests tended by lone parents in Sweden') containing the latest National Institute for Clinical Excellence (NICE) guidance was next. These always seem to concern things we've been managing perfectly well all these years, but which suddenly need managing in a completely different way because a load of academics who've never spent a day in general practice say so.

In this particular case, it was the latest diabetes guidance.

The Standard Operating Procedure for this used to be:

> Diet
> Then drug A
> Then drug B
> Then drug A+B
> Then insulin.
> Job done.

Admittedly, things have got a little more complicated since the pharma companies have had the audacity to develop new drugs. But now we're left with this low-sugar dog's breakfast:

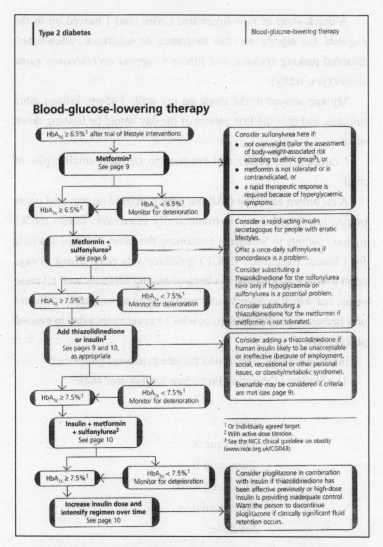

Blood-glucose-lowering therapy

HbA$_{1c}$ ≥ 6.5%[1] after trial of lifestyle interventions

Metformin[2]
See page 9

Consider sulfonylurea here if:
- not overweight (tailor the assessment of body-weight-associated risk according to ethnic group[3]), or
- metformin is not tolerated or is contraindicated, or
- a rapid therapeutic response is required because of hyperglycaemic symptoms.

HbA$_{1c}$ ≥ 6.5%[1]

HbA$_{1c}$ < 6.5%[1]
Monitor for deterioration

Metformin + sulfonylurea[2]
See page 9

Consider a rapid-acting insulin secretagogue for people with erratic lifestyles.

Offer a once-daily sulfonylurea if concordance is a problem.

Consider substituting a thiazolidinedione for the sulfonylurea here only if hypoglycaemia on sulfonylurea is a potential problem.

Consider substituting a thiazolidinedione for the metformin if metformin is not tolerated.

HbA$_{1c}$ ≥ 7.5%[1]

HbA$_{1c}$ < 7.5%[1]
Monitor for deterioration

Add thiazolidinedione or insulin[2]
See pages 9 and 10, as appropriate

Consider adding a thiazolidinedione if human insulin likely to be unacceptable or ineffective (because of employment, social, recreational or other personal issues, or obesity/metabolic syndrome).

Exenatide may be considered if criteria are met (see page 9).

HbA$_{1c}$ ≥ 7.5%[1]

HbA$_{1c}$ < 7.5%[1]
Monitor for deterioration

Insulin + metformin + sulfonylurea[2]
See page 10

[1] Or individually agreed target.
[2] With active dose titration.
[3] See the NICE clinical guideline on obesity (www.nice.org.uk/CG043).

HbA$_{1c}$ ≥ 7.5%[1]

HbA$_{1c}$ < 7.5%[1]
Monitor for deterioration

Increase insulin dose and intensify regimen over time
See page 10

Consider pioglitazone in combination with insulin if thiazolidinedione has been effective previously or high-dose insulin is providing inadequate control. Warn the person to discontinue pioglitazone if clinically significant fluid retention occurs.

It makes my eyes bleed just to look at it.

Bear in mind this is just one of 19 pages in the document, and that this document is – no kidding – the 'Quick reference guide'. The *full* guide is the size of a telephone directory.

Will I read it? No.

Will it matter? No, because by the time I do, it will all have changed again, anyway.

Now, what's this? A postcard from Kelly Jupe who is on holiday in Marbella with her boyfriend:

> *Dear Doc Cop!! Having a gr8 time (and using plenty of Factor 30 and watching my units lol!!!!!)*
> *Just a quick note to say that I done what you said and took them pills but I've still got that like irritating pain in my neck???*
> *Kelly xxx*

Thanks, Kelly – I know exactly how you feel.

A complaint from a patient about something or other – not quite mad enough to warrant a place on the common room notice board, though – and some stuff from the PCT about my prescribing data and my 'balanced scorecard'.* I frowned: most of the PCT crud gets diverted to the practice manager, Jane Carstone. I put it to one side, looking forward to passing it on later with my broadest smile.

Some guff from the Benefits Agency, a few requests for information from employers and charitable institutions and a solicitor's letter:

> *'Further to our previous correspondence, Mrs Grimwig has informed our office that the flat immediately below hers is currently occupied by a drug dealer. Can you confirm that this would have a detrimental effect on her health?'*

No. In fact it might even save the NHS some money if she were to deal direct. (And that will be £37.50, thanks.)

Finally, the usual survey – this week's came from BigPharmCo and invited me to indicate whether I would consider using a 'new but not yet established' drug for the treatment of patients with something or other. The survey will be followed up with invitations to 'educational' meetings at ritzy restaurants at BigPharmCo's expense. But I don't much like surveys, or ritzy restaurants, so I scrunched it up in a ball and aimed it at the wastepaper bin on the other side of the room; it bounced off the rim and joined the other thirty or so which were lying at various distances from the target.

I looked at the clock: 7:59am. Just time to clear them all up before I opened the door to Mrs Chuffey and her terrible thrush.

* You might be wondering what a 'balanced scorecard' is, and what relevance it has to my performance as a doctor. Me too. The BS is an intensely bureaucratic and obsessively box-ticking way of ranking GP practices in order that those where the doctors are trying to kill you/discriminating against you/generally failing to comply with Department of Health diktats can be identified and punished. A fuller explanation, running to around 10,000 words of jargon, can be found at the NHS primary care commissioning website (if you are at all interested).

CANCER WAITING LISTS

OUR local graffiti artistes had been hard at it when I arrived for work at the virus/human interface yesterday, after a pleasant weekend away in the honeyed charm of the Cotswolds.

The following conversation had taken place on our building, in alternate and indelible black and silver marker pen.

Fuck u TOO, Knobhead! Chuzzlewit rulez
Who YOU callin a Nobhead?
U no hoo I mean, knobface!
Kyle Chuzlewit is a knobhead
Fuk u knob breath
KYLE CHUZLEWIT = GAYYYYY!!!!!

Most invigorating: Banksy, eat your vandalising little heart out.

Inside, I met a distressed young mum, Ms Pinch.

She was 22 and had been suffering for a while with bloody diarrhoea.

By that I don't mean simply that she was exasperated by it; I mean it really *was* bloody. The problem had been continuing on and off for some time, was getting worse, and now she was losing weight. She was embarrassed and she was frightened – not least because she'd read in some magazine that this was among the symptoms of bowel cancer.

I didn't think for a moment she had bowel cancer. What I did think she had was inflammatory bowel disease – specifically, either ulcerative colitis or Crohn's disease, both unpleasant, both of 'idiopathic' or unknown cause and both quite capable of making a patient feel pretty ill.

She needed to be seen at the hospital quickly to confirm my diagnosis in order that treatment – industrial doses of steroids – could begin as soon as possible. She'd already left it a while before coming to see me, and this is one of those things which really shouldn't be left.

As with Charlie Darnay and his ME, and Mr Marley and his dodgy shoulder, there was a time when I could simply have phoned my favourite gastroenterologist, had a quick chat about Ms Pinch, and she'd have been seen within a day or two.

Now? Oh, dear me, no – that would never do. She has to enter the 'system'.

That was when the problems started, and they were caused by the government's famous cancer waiting list pledge.

A while back, Labour announced that 'cancer patients' would be referred to a specialist within two weeks of presenting to their GP.

Well, it made a great headline (headlines plural, actually – the pledge has been regularly wheeled out and repeated over the years).

At first glance it doesn't look a bad idea. People with cancer will be seen within a fortnight – who'd be against a target like that?

Me, for starters.

The trouble with things like this is that they are motivated entirely by sound bite politics – its only useful purpose was that it allowed Gordon Brown to stand up at a podium, make a pledge and then dare the Tories not to support it.

What people like Mr Brown either don't understand or pretend not to know is that we hardly ever send 'people with cancer' to a specialist.

Sometimes we do, sure – and in those cases, we could do with having our patients seen that day, never mind a fortnight hence.

But mostly we send people up with symptoms which *might* be compatible with cancer but *might* be lots of others things as well. The fact is, they often don't need to be seen within two weeks – in some cases, it might surprise you to know, even if they *are* cancers.

Since the two week rule was decreed by the bureaucrats in Whitehall, the hospital clinics are stuffed with query cancers which don't really need seeing quickly and the knock-on effect of this is there are lots of patients with *non*-cancerous problems who *do* need seeing quickly – people like Ms Pinch – whom we can't get seen quickly because, you guessed it, all the clinics are full of query cancers.

What to do?

I could be dishonest and claim that I *thought* she might have cancer, but I didn't think she had so it wouldn't have been professional (some GPs do play games like this and they get found out very quickly).

It was tempting to send her up as an 'acute admission' – an 'emergency', in other words. Then she'd get sorted out in two shakes of a colonoscope. But, again, I'd get a bollocking for 'abusing the system'.

So instead of a nice natter on the phone with the gastroenterologist, I had to resort to pleading, cajoling and shouting to get anything done – knowing full well that the appointment I eventually secured would probably be cancelled anyway.

The other side of this invidious coin is that once you trumpet these pledges at your political rallies, you create expectations in people. Sometimes, you create expectations in people who ought to know better. Recently, I read that GPs are 'complacent' about cancer referrals. Says who? Professor Steve Field – the generally excellent chairman of the Royal College of General Practitioners, no less. Apparently, a new report has found GPs fail to refer a significant number of cancers under the two week rule. To which my response is, if you take the number of GPs in the country (around 41,000), multiply by the numbers of patient interactions and divide by the fact that cancer doesn't always look like or act as the textbooks say it should, then of course some will be missed (and some things that turn out not to be cancer will be referred).

Complacency, though? I don't think so. We all live in fear of missing the Big C, but that doesn't make it any easier to sift the pathological needle from the polysymptomatic haystack.

The simple stats hide the complex truth. Politicians and journalists could be forgiven for thinking that medicine is black and white. They can't understand the nuances which we have to agonise over – the patient diagnosed with diverticular disease who presents a year later with more diarrhoea, the bloating woman whose chronic anxiety would reach breakdown point if she's investigated, the elderly patient unwilling to pursue the rectal bleed which is probably just piles anyway… plus there's the fact that cancer doesn't always oblige with text-book symptoms because the mitotic process – by which cancer cells divide and grow – hates GPs, too, and wants to make us look lazy and incompetent. This is real life practice and it has the potential to screw up patient lives *and* our referral stats. Being a GP, Prof Field understands this. And being our figurehead, you'd like to think he'd point it out.

Of course, we could all take the easy route and refer urgently any patient with even the slightest hint of a whiff of a suspicion of something vaguely neoplastic. That way, our arses would be covered, and all the GP-knockers would presumably be happy. Until they discover that the two week wait has morphed into two years – which would result in accusations of defensive medicine. At least that would make a change from complacency!

REBECCA BAGNET, AGAIN

I WAS TOYING WITH the idea of checking my favourite searches on eBay during my coffee break when the phone rang. It was Gordon, receptionist extraordinaire. Even as he spoke I heard the voice of Jilted John in my head.

'Er, Tony…'

Memo to self: *Ask Jane to remind Reception staff to refer to us as 'Doctor This' and 'Doctor That' when patients are within earshot.*

'Er, Gordon…?'

'Er, Tony, would you be all right about seeing a 15-year-old girl without her parents as a Book on the Day walk-in and wait thingy? She says she's run out of insulin.'

'Who is it?'

'Er, Becca Bagnet.'

Around half an hour later, she shambled into my office in full-on emo regalia. Dyed black asymmetric hair, enough eyeliner to sink the ocean-going variety and a selection of Oxfam shop bangles adorning a pair of painfully thin forearms.

'Rebecca.'

'Doc.'

'How are things?'

'Crap. Same as always.'

'Mum and dad OK?'

'Guess so.'

'What's with the diabetes thing?'

'S'alright.'

'That's not what I've been hearing.'

'Like what?'

'Like you've been waking up in Casualty rather a lot recently. Is there something particularly tasty about hospital sugar lumps these days?'

'They don't do sugar lumps. They do injections.'

'I know. It was a joke.'

'Ha ha.'

'And these injections… you usually end up needing them after your friends have tried the sugar lump and/or glucose liquid thing, and you haven't come round.'

I pulled a random selection of her casualty cards onto the PC screen... blood glucose levels less than 3mmol/litre, brought in by paramedics or by concerned friends, drifting in and out of consciousness, revived by an injection of glucagon (the hormone the body uses to release stored glucose from the liver into the bloodstream). One A&E report mentioned vodka, another mentioned Bacardi and a third referred to a possible seizure *en route* in the ambulance.

'Do your mum and dad know that you're here?'

'I can look after myself can't I?'

'Well, judging by these hospital reports, no, you can't.'

'You're as bad as they are. Do I get my Lantus and Humalog or not?'

Lantus and Humalog are types of insulin, obviously.

'What about some finger-prickers and testing sticks to check your blood sugar?'

'Got plenty.'

Which meant that she wasn't using them. Type 1 diabetics like Rebecca are people whose insulin-producing cells have been destroyed; they are treated by delivering replacement insulin via injections or a pump, and ensuring they eat a healthy diet and take plenty of exercise. They need to adjust their insulin doses in line with their blood glucose level, and this is determined by pricking a finger to obtain blood, checking the reading and then dosing according to the size of the next meal, the amount of exercise planned etc etc.

I leaned back in my chair and looked at her for a moment. She stared back, defiantly.

'Right,' I said. 'Here's a prescription. But I'm not resetting your repeat medication request slip until I see the results of these blood tests and a note from the Diabetic Day Care Centre saying you've been in for a pep talk.'

I handed over the prescription and a pathology test card. Blood pressure 90/58. Body Mass Index 17. Kate Moss eat your heart out. What it is to be young.

MARTHA

GPs love to depict themselves as workers at the coalface, toiling heroically in the pits of pathology for the benefit of society. In truth, it often feels more like the misery of war than the dignity of labour. Which is why, whenever I imagine a TV version of primary care, the image that springs to mind is *M*A*S*H** – remember that?

I'd be Hawkeye, obviously, Dr Emma would be a doctory version of Hotlips Houlihan and – especially on a Monday morning – the punters would be the forces of North Korea.

As for Radar, who had superhuman hearing and could detect incoming choppers before anyone else: no contest. That would be Martha Bardell, my aforementioned medical secretary.

She's supposed to be responsible for secretarial tasks such as typing letters, fielding queries from patients and arranging meetings. Which she does, very well. But that's not all. Not by a long way.

Martha is the oracle. My second brain. My guardian angel who covers my cock-ups, remembers what I forget and clears up the mess I make. Without her, I would be hopeless and helpless. Like Radar, she seems to know everything that's going on, often before it's happened. And she's a treasure-trove of useful information – if you want the number of any of the local consultants' private secretaries, the waiting time for any clinic you'd care to mention or the exact, rather than approximate, date of your wedding anniversary, she has it stored in her memory.

I suspect many GPs have their own particular Martha. In which case, they'll recognise the following interaction.

'Ah, Martha, I saw Mr Heathfield's wife about his memory problems yesterday and I couldn't recall where…'

'The memory assessment team's now based just outside of town. In the community clinic.'

'Of course. So…'

'Tuesdays and Thursdays. In the afternoon. They'll need a referral letter.'

'Of course. But…'

'I know, he shouldn't drive. And his wife doesn't, not since her stroke. So, bus number 56. From the stop on the high street. Every half hour.'

'Excellent. Sorry, what's…?'

Martha has just handed me a piece of paper.

'The referral letter for you to sign.'

She's brilliant at the really serious stuff, too – like this.

'Martha, we have a crisis.'

'We did, Dr Copperfield, but we don't now.'

'We don't?'

'No. Because I bought more Hob Nobs this morning. Two packs chocolate, two packs plain.'

I give a quizzical look.

'Your waist size has just gone up to 36. You were talking to Dr Patel about it the other day. Something about insulin resistance. So you've got the option – choccy or no choccy. Plus they were buy one, get one free.'

Most of my working life involves people trying to dump work on me or shirk responsibility. Community nurses who say things like, 'Dr Copperfield, Mrs Sleary's foot has gone blue. Just thought I'd let you know.' Consultants who copy to me the grossly abnormal results of blood tests they've arranged 'For your information', when they really mean, 'For your action.' 'Shared-care protocols' – designed to divvy up the work of a complex case between the specialist and the GP – which are, in reality, 'Shifted care protocols', with everything landing in my lap. In this context, Martha is a breath of fresh air: someone who presents me with solutions rather than problems.

But today, she really excelled herself.

'Dr Copperfield, I was typing the agenda for next Monday's practice meeting,' she began, walking into the common room while I was having a coffee. I hurriedly put the chocolate Hob Nob back in the tin and rummaged for the plain version. 'And I checked through the minutes of the last meeting. I noticed under "Action" that you were nominated to have a meeting with the staff of Rosemount Gardens Retirement Home. Together with the community nurses? To sort out the number of visit requests you're getting and some prescribing issues?'

Bugger. I'd completely forgotten. I'm supposed to 'feedback' in the practice pow-wow.

'So I hope you don't mind, but I contacted the home manager and a couple of the nurses. They're coming over at lunchtime today.'

'Ah…' I began. 'The only thing is…'

'I've rescheduled your tutorial for tomorrow,' she said.

'Right, but…'

'There's a weekly breakdown of visit requests for the last six months in your pigeon hole, with copies for the others,' she said.

'Excellent, but…'

'And I've ordered lunch. Sandwiches. With no tomato.'

I hate tomato. But I think I love Martha. She's wasted running meetings. She should be running the NHS.

MR PICKWICK

EVEN MORE GRAFFITI on the exterior of the building, now.

This time:

> *Kyle Chuzlewit is a benda*
> *Fuk u u bastad*
> *Kyle Chuzlewit + John Chivery = 1 item*
> *Fuk u knobhead!*

I wondered if Mr Chuzzlewit was one of our patients: I checked, and it turned out he wasn't. He obviously just likes hanging around the surgery taunting, and being taunted by, his peers.

Mid way through what was proving to be an even less interesting morning than usual, up popped Mr Pickwick: mid-50s, on his third marriage, doting father of two youngish children.

He was the archetypal 'Diamond Geezer' – more front than Southend and more gold on each hand than Mrs Copperfield has in the whole of her jewellery box. It contrasted nicely with the nicotine stains from the perma-fag he held, sniper style in his palm.

'Tell you what, doc,' he said. 'Sort this cough out, will you?'

Ah, such a diagnostic challenge, and so early in the day.

'OK,' I said. 'You've got a cough. You've been smoking roll-ups for as long as I've known you – which is nigh on 20 years – and you've got a cough. Make it interesting: three minutes, starting now.'

'I've got this cough.'

Then, as most men do when they're trying to describe a symptom, he ran out of ideas. Time for a little 'direct questioning'.

This is what good doctors aren't supposed to do, these days. We're supposed to settle back and listen, rapt, while you relate your medical history with such astounding clarity that the diagnosis falls out at our feet like a shoplifted CD at the checkout. Real world doctors resort to 'To Direct Questioning' when patients are unable or unwilling to tell us what's wrong. So if you forget your lines while telling me about a headache, for example, I'll ask you what it feels like, what time of day it's most likely to come on and whether it comes on suddenly or gradually, what else happens at the same time, and whether anything seems to make it better. It's the answers to questions like these, rather than the pantomime cocking around with blood pressure machines and ophthalmoscopes, that tell me whether you're describing a symptom of overwork, migraine or a brain tumour.

Back to Mr Pickwick. TDQ, he admitted that he'd had the cough for about six weeks, it was usually dry and hacking and painful, and that it hurt when he took a deep breath (especially on the right side). Once or twice he'd noticed some blood on the Kleenex after his ritual morning hawk-up.

I sat him up on the exam couch and listened to his chest. With each breath he took I heard a faint crunching noise as if he was eating dry Rice Krispies in time with his breathing.

'Are you getting short of breath these days?'

'Now you mention it, doc, I am a bit. Walking the dog's getting a bit too much for me. The odd thing is, I've lost half a stone in the last couple of months.'

'How have you managed that?'

'I dunno, really. It's just kind of fell off me.'

I lay him down flat on the couch, loosened the belt (fake designer) of his jeans (genuine George at ASDA) and prodded around his abdomen.

'Take a really deep breath for me?'

As he did so, I felt the edge of his liver pushing against my fingertips.

'You much of a drinker?'

'Well, you know me, doc. Life and soul. Had a major night last weekend, my big sister's Ruby wedding anniversary.'

'I'll bet you had a curry, eh?'

'What?'

'Ruby. Ruby Murray. Curry.'

'Very droll, doc. You ought to get a job writing comedy.'

'Well?'

'Well what?'

'Curry?'

He thought for a moment, screwing up his face as he did so. Then he let out a sigh. 'Do you know what, doc,' he said. 'I can't bleeding remember. Ain't that weird – it's only a few days ago. Anyway, what's the verdict? Will I live?'

'I'm pretty sure you've got pleurisy. Something's inflaming the edge of your lung and it's swollen up so it drags along the inside of your chest wall as you breathe. What you need is a chest X-ray and some antibiotics. Come and see me again next Wednesday.'

I employed my mastery of the computerised appointment system to book him in to a slot labelled 'BOOK <u>ON THE DAY ONLY</u> – ACCESS TARGETS MATTER!'

'No, they bloody don't,' I said under my breath.

There was something about Mr Pickwick that worried me, and that's what mattered.

LYING BASTARDS

EVERY TUESDAY LUNCHTIME, our key practice staff – doctors, nurses, medical sec Martha, practice manager Staffelführer Jane Carstone, occasionally the head receptionist Mrs Peggotty – assemble for an 'educational' meeting in the seminar room, lured by the prospect of some free sandwiches from Morrisons and a satsuma.

The format never varies and rarely does my sense of *ennui*. Whoever drew the short straw for the week presents an 'interesting' case or prepares a sleep-inducing Power Point presentation on a gripping topic such as 'New developments in leg ulcer dressings' or 'Chilblains – the patient's experience'.

This week we were expecting a real treat, a session on 'Holistic care of the elderly housebound patient', but the nurse expected to lead the discussion had booked the day off as sick leave several weeks ago and apparently no one had noticed.

We all sat twiddling our thumbs, sighing and wondering what to do. To break the ice I asked if anybody had seen a recent survey that showed that 85 per cent of people still trusted their doctors to tell the truth. That makes us just about the most trusted group of people there is. Weird!

The silence was broken by a snort from the corner. It was Sami Patel. 'Never mind *us* telling *them* the truth,' he said. 'What about the bastards telling *us* the truth once in a while?'

'Now then, Dr Patel,' said Frau Carstone. 'Our patients may be liars, but they are not bastards.'

'Actually, quite a lot of them are, Jane,' I said. 'Technically-speaking, I mean.'

'Look,' said Sami. 'I realise that if I repeated this outside these four walls I'd be in danger of destroying thousands of beautiful doctor-patient relationships, but do we really trust our patients? The truthful answer is no.'

'I don't think any of my patients lie to me,' said Dr Emma, drawing an approving glance from Jane P.

'Well, you don't get to deal with any of the local junkies* for a start,' said Sami. 'Half the dogs round here must live on methadone prescriptions, considering the number which get mysteriously chewed up and need replacing. You ask a patient if he's been taking his blood pressure pills properly, and it will be all, "Oh, yes doctor!" And I'm like, "Well that's weird, because your repeat prescription hasn't been collected since last October".'

'I'm the same at the dentist, to be fair,' I said, performing some essential research into Hob Nob dunking. '"Have you been flossing regularly?" "Of course I have!" *Since yesterday*. It's more about not wanting to hurt peoples' feelings – especially people with a drill in your mouth.'

'I think it's about how you ask the question,' said Dr Emma. 'I don't ask if they're taking their blood pressure pills, I ask, "How often do you forget to take them?" It's about being non-threatening, Sami. They're happy to admit to missing a dose now and then.'

Silence reigned again for a moment or two, as Sami digested this novel piece of fluffy yet devious feminine psychology.

'Anyway, don't get me started on bloody asthmatics,' he said, finally.

There was a murmur of agreement. If any pathology particularly breeds pathological fibbers, it's asthma. Research has proven that most of the self-monitoring that asthmatics document is, in fact, fabricated: all those Peak Flow Readings, neatly entered into their Peak Flow Diaries, over a period of six months, and *always with the same pen*.

'They'll insist that their inhaler technique is perfect,' said Sami, 'but then they blow when they ought to be sucking and you realise they might as well be squirting it under their armpits for all the good it'll be doing them.'

'No wonder they're breathless when they make their appointments,' said Jane. 'They're terrified they'll get one with you.'

By now, Sami was on a roll. 'Cardiac patients who insist they're taking their statins, when we know more than half of them knock the drugs on the head within a year. Boozers who smell of alcohol at ten in the morning but swear they only have a couple of pints one night a week and maybe a few at the weekend. Callers exaggerating every tiny little problem to try and wangle an unnecessary home visit... aaaarrrgggh! Do you want me to go on?'

'The thing is,' I said, 'if 85 per cent of the population think we tell the truth, that means that 15 per cent don't. Those ones don't trust us at all.'

'Like I say,' said Sami, triumphantly. 'Bastards.'

* Apologies: I meant Community Based Drug Misuse Assessment and Progress Supervision Service users (vulnerable).

LATER THAT SAME DAY

OF COURSE, DOCTORS lie too – once in a while. It's all about how you define 'lie'.

In fact, later that same day I began psyching myself up for a Great White Shark of a Big White Lie.

I was still grinning at the memory of Sami's indignant outburst when Mr Pickwick's test results arrived in my inbox.

At that moment, the grin froze.

The chest x-ray I ordered last week showed a huge tumour in his right lung. Immediately, I suspected that it had already seeded secondary deposits throughout his body to account for his weight loss, liver enlargement and memory lapses.

As soon as I saw it, I visualised myself sending him on his way to the oncology department with a firm handshake and my best wishes for a future he almost certainly doesn't have. I would refer him for further tests. There'd be a CT scan, a biopsy, some blood tests and possibly some exploratory surgery that would really amount to nothing more than a premature autopsy.

This is a kind of lie, I think: by ordering this extra work, I'm giving him hope of a cure, telling him that 'something can be done', when in fact I know, deep down, that his chances of surviving six months are no better than 50/50 and that he's already seen his last Christmas.

It's not a blatant untruth. I'm trying to give my patient some hope – hope that, in all probability, will turn out to be false. And of course there is a tiny outside chance that I could be wrong. The actor Stewart Granger used to tell a story about a chest X-ray he had that showed what appeared to be a large tumour, and how he got the 'few weeks to live' chat from his doctor. In fact, the mass turned out to be benign; he had a cannonball-shaped cavity in his lung, presumably from childhood TB, and he'd got a fungal infection growing within the cavity. What were the chances? About the same as being struck by lightning twice.

Nobody, apart from Mr Pickwick, his immediate family and his Labrador, will be happier than I if he turns out to have something equally unlikely and is left with nothing more than a story that he can dine out on for years.

But I know that after the biopsy result comes through it will be time to sit down and talk about palliative care and, if he can face up to it, what he wants me to organise when the time comes. Home or hospice? Burial or cremation? Cancer Research or flowers?

There are other ways in which we might bend the truth to help you.

Doctors have always known that our patients' recoveries depend just as much on the quality of the doctor-patient interaction – or to use the technical term, the bullshitting – as they do on the actual treatment.

If I hand over a prescription with a hearty, 'This stuff's marvellous, took it myself once, it had me back on my feet in no time at all!' it's been proven that it'll work better than a much more potent prescription issued with a wordless sigh. (I've never taken the drug at all – that's the lie.) Conversely, 'You might as well give these a try but I'm not promising anything' could well undermine a really 'powerful' drug (not least, I suppose, because the chances of the patient actually having the prescription made up would be reduced).

The old and familiar 'I think it's just a virus' line is kind of a fib, too. It's our get-out when we haven't the faintest idea what's really going on, but know that the patient likes to think we do, and will gain comfort and reassurance from diagnosis. Of course, it often really *is* just a virus, but while we're waiting to find out, we do the worrying rather than you.

And then there's the 'I'm more certain than I really am' fib. Sick people get better more quickly and cope better with their illness if they are given a definite diagnosis – even one that is made up on the spot by translating their presenting symptoms into cod Latin. It's a psychological thing. If you think I don't know what's really wrong with you – and a huge part of my day-to-day work involves dealing with diagnostic uncertainty – then you'll be less likely to take my advice, even if it's just to wait and see and not worry too much. Famously, one family doctor, on hearing his favourite hypochondriac describe 'a burning pain down my right leg whenever I burp' diagnosed 'eructative dextro-sciatic neuralgia'. All that really means is a trapped nerve with the symptoms exacerbated by belching, but the medical-sounding words reassured the patient that he was in good hands. In much the same way, if I tell a chap with muscle stiffness and inflammation that he has 'fibromyositis', he'll happily slap on lotions that have little direct effect and will recover more quickly than if I just tell him he's pulled a muscle.

Some patients respond to placebos even when they *know* they are in a controlled trial with a chance of getting sham treatment. For a long time, these folks were considered by proper doctors (like me) to be a few ham sandwiches short of a picnic – to be pitied, along with those considered good subjects for hypnosis or particularly receptive to Reiki or manipulation of their auras and bank balances. But now there is a rational explanation: recent research indicates that placebo-responders are not gullible fools after all. Instead, they are just better than most people at synthesising the neurotransmitter dopamine, found in the parts of the brain concerned with desire and reward. Apparently, they just want to get better more than the rest of us, and so they do.

It all reminds me of the credo that kept me going through medical school: 'Everything I learn will be proven wrong some day.'

Unfortunately, as far as Mr Pickwick is concerned, that day has not yet arrived for lung cancer.

LUCIE THE REGISTRAR

I SPENT A DAY last week with our new registrar, Lucie Manette – Sami Patel's tall blonde with 'bags of potential'.

Unfortunately, while she looks as described – and is a charming person to boot – her potential, at least as a doctor, is another thing altogether. In fact, she reminded me once again why I hope one day to die under a speeding bus and be thus spared a lingering death under the care of the next generation of medics.

To become a GP, you do your standard five years at university gaining a degree – the Bachelor of Medicine and Bachelor of Surgery. You then do a further five years' postgraduate training – two 'foundation years', usually involving hospital posts, then two years of hospital jobs geared toward general practice, like obstetrics and gynaecology, paediatrics and A&E and a final year working solely in general practice as a 'registrar'.

You might think that after nine whole years in the incubator to date, Lucie would be guaranteed to emerge from the process absolutely chock-full of medical knowledge. She ought to be crammed with information, bursting with diagnoses and positively leaking technical expertise from her overstuffed cerebrum.

Sadly, she isn't.

Don't get me wrong. There are certain medical students who you can tell from day one should never deal with sentient beings. Instead, they should be confined in small spaces where they can peer into microscopes and send out emails, or be forced to become anaesthetists, who are mainly employed to laugh at surgeons' jokes. Lucie isn't like that. She seems a nice, bright young woman, and she's terrifically keen, but she appears to know almost nothing about medicine; in this she is like almost every other trainee doc I've come across in recent years.

It's not her fault – it's all about pendulums (or is it pendula?).

When I started training back in the 1970s, information was king. Doctors *knew* stuff. We rote-learned reams of body parts, diseases, symptoms and therapeutics. One textbook was actually called *The Book of Medical Lists*, and it doesn't need any more explaining than that. Another – our bible – was *Hutchison's Clinical Methods*, an offensive weapon of a tome which was full of tiresome detail: *This is a patient's head/knee/elbow/shoulder/neck/etc, and this is how you examine the given bit.*

It wasn't perfect – for a start off, lots of the things we learned as 'fact' turned out to be nonsense – but we had a foundation level of basic, practical knowledge upon which we could build once we started out in the world.

Unfortunately, some people felt that medicine was too academic, doctors were too authoritarian and they couldn't talk to patients. So the pendulum swung: all the wet, soppy guff they used to knock out of you at medical school, they started trying to stuff more of it *in*. Chiefly, they went massive on communication. The result: Lucie and all the thousands of other new recruits have a *fantastic* bedside manner. They could tell you you had terminal cancer and six hours to live and you'd thank them. They are *world* class at talking to patients. Unfortunately, they have next to nothing worth saying. (It's not just me saying this – a recent *British Medical Journal* survey of consultants and specialist registrars in two teaching hospitals found students were not 'well prepared for clinical life' because they 'lack core knowledge and skills'. Nothing too important you understand, just stuff like prescribing and how to manage ill people.)

As part of her training, Lucie will be seeing some patients alone (not unresponsive children with a rash that won't fade, or people asking for Herceptin), and then discussing the issues afterwards with me.

The first case we talked through was that of a chap in his 50s who hobbled in after twisting his knee playing football with his grandson.

'Tell me about Mr Bazzard,' I said. 'What did you do?'

'Well, he was experiencing pain in the knee, so I thought I'd order an MRI scan for him,' she said.

'OK, back up a sec,' I said. 'When you examined the knee, what did you find wrong with it?'

She looked at me blankly. 'When I *examined* it?'

'Yes. You must have examined it? Poked it and prodded it and felt about a bit?'

'Well, I *looked* at it,' she said, dubiously. 'It looked a bit swollen.'

'Did you test the ligaments? Did you check for cartilage damage? Did you look for any effusion?'

'Erm,' she said. 'I didn't do orthopaedics.'

'I can't believe they don't just teach you this stuff as a matter of course,' I said. 'Examining a knee is about as basic as it gets. You'll see hundreds, no thousands, of knees in your career, Lucie. Laying hands on them will often locate the damage and rule out the need for an MRI.'

'Why would I want to rule out an MRI?'

'MRIs are expensive, for one thing. For another, there aren't that many of the machines. If everyone in the country who ever trips up and falls over gets sent for a scan, think of the people with serious problems who actually need an MRI who will have to wait. Plus, if you can reassure Mr Bazzard there and then that it's nothing major, and all he really needs to do is take some ibuprofen and rest it for a few days, why put him to the inconvenience of having to go over to the hospital three weeks on Wednesday to pay six quid to park and wait for an hour, when the knee will have cleared up by then anyway?'

I know this sounds a bit 'in my day', but the fact is that MRI is on the same continuum as x-rays, bloods and biopsies. They are all, to a lesser or greater extent, expensive, invasive and time-consuming and if they are not needed they should not be done.

'OK,' she said. 'Can you show me how to examine a knee, then?'

'Show you how to examine a bloody knee?' I said. '*Jeez!* And for the tutorial after that? Which way round to hold a sodding tongue depressor?'

At least, that's what I should have said. But I didn't, because I'm used to this kind of thing by now. Instead, I said, wearily, 'Sure. Now, tell me about Mr Pecksniff.'

Mr Pecksniff is an elderly resident of the Rosemount Gardens Retirement Home. Lucie had seen him earlier that day, and he turned out to offer great scope for a 'Case-based Discussion', as we're supposed to call it. He was a bit demented, he'd been losing weight and his relatives were pushing for him to have artificial feeding. There are lots of nice points here – some medical (why is he losing weight?) and others ethical (essentially, when can doctors force-feed a grown man if he can't give consent?)

'Er…' said Lucie.

'Just talk me through the issues.'

There was a long silence. Eventually, she spoke. 'Well… I… erm…'

'OK,' I said. 'Do we know why he's losing weight?'

'Well… I… erm…'

'Should we investigate?'

'Er…'

'Does he have capacity?'

'Umm…'

'What happens when the staff try to feed him?'

'Er…'

'What do you think the relatives are hoping to achieve?'

'Umm…'

I took a big breath and decided to try one more time.

'Even if you don't know the answers, do you know what the key issues are here?'

Silence.

'I don't know the protocols for this sort of situation,' she said, finally.

Standardised 'protocols' in medicine are supposed to promote high and uniform practice. Instead, they're creating in young doctors an epidemic of brain paralysis. Take away the comfort blanket of the protocol and they're lost.

'There *is* no protocol for this,' I said. 'You have to *think*. For yourself.'

I should stress again, I'm not saying everything was better in the old days, but at least you learnt – on a steep and scary curve – about medicine and about taking responsibility. Trainees nowadays are over-supervised to the point that they appear to spend more time having 'assessments' than they do seeing patients and learning to think and act on their feet. And if you don't have that level of responsibility I reckon you can't maintain a decent level of interest, either. Which is why, when I ask Lucie how you treat the funny lumps on a patients' legs that she'd correctly – and amazingly – identified as erythema nodosum, she didn't know.

'We had a patient with this at the hospital,' she said. 'But I went off duty before they got to the treatment bit.'

I looked at my clock. 'Let's have a break for a coffee?' I said. 'Afterwards you can sit in and watch me. I think it would help.'

PROTECTING PEOPLE FROM THEMSELVES

I WALKED IN to the Common Room as Sami Patel was leaving.

'Copperfield, you sly old dog!' he said, by way of a greeting. 'It hasn't taken you long to get into bed with young Lucie, has it? Figuratively-speaking, I mean.'

'If you want to take her off my hands, be my guest,' I said.

'Great bedside manner, no practical skills or knowledge?' he said, with a fair stab at a sympathetic face. 'The usual story? You sound like my old man. "Young doctors, dey hev assoluttly no idea, Samit! *You* hev assoluttly no idea!" He must be about your age, my dad. Actually, maybe a touch younger.'

'He sounds pretty switched on,' I said. 'You must take after your mum?'

'Joking apart, though,' said Sami, 'he's right, innee? All this bollocks about doctors being too authoritarian... there's a link between knowing stuff and being authoritarian. Mechanics know how to fix cars. Your alternator's fucked, 200 quid, ready at four-thirty. People don't complain that they're authoritarian, or that they don't break it to you gently, and ask how you *feel* about your alternator. They just hand over the 200 squids and thank their lucky stars they're still on the road.'

Just then, Lucie appeared to collect her coffee. Sami held the door open for her – slyly looking her up and down as he did so, and grinning like a Bollywood megastar.

'Hi Lucie,' he said. 'How's it going with Tony? If you're struggling with the generation gap, feel free to slide down to my room where we practice slightly more up-to-date medicine.'

'It's... I'll be fine, thanks,' she said.

'Well, you know where I am,' said Sami. 'By the way... that stuff about alternators, I don't know if you overheard? We were talking about Tony's Nissan. Mine's the silver Porsche. It's certainly not fucked. It's bloody nearly brand new! Laters!'

With that, he was gone.

'What was that all about?' said Lucie.

'Nothing that a good shrink couldn't handle,' I said.

Back in my consulting room a few minutes later, we saw Mr Bates, a builder who kept collapsing.

'It's weird,' he said. 'Three times now I've ended up on the floor not knowing how I got there.'

After a little digging, it became clear that these were more than simple faints.

'I think I know what the problem is, Mr Bates,' I said. 'You're suffering fits. We're going to need to get this checked out.'

'OK, doc,' he said. 'Can you sign me off on the sick?'

'Are you working at the moment?' I said.

'No, there ain't no work around at the minute. But if I can get on the sick rather than the dole, that would be better.'

'Well, I guess it would be difficult for you to sort out a job while you're having fits. Wouldn't be a great idea to be perched on some scaffolding…'

'Oh, cheers doc,' he said. 'Only, I've been wanting to get on the sick for ages.'

'…so I'll sign the forms for you. Can I ask, how did you get here today?'

'I drove.'

'Ah.'

'Ah?'

'Yes. You see, on the upside – from your point of view – you can't work because of your condition, but on the downside you also can't *drive* because of your condition.'

'What d'you mean, I can't drive?' he said, a note of indignation creeping into his voice.

'If you're not safe carrying a hod or walking down the stairs, how can you be safe behind the wheel of a tonne of metal doing 50 miles an hour? You're going to have to inform the DVLA of your condition and take yourself off the road for the time being, I'm afraid.'

'No fucking way,' he said. 'Excuse my French, miss, but no way. I need my bleeding car to get to the pub, to the footie, to get down the bookies, to get down my mate's house, to take the missus to the shops… no fucking way.'

'Firstly,' I said. 'Please don't swear at me. Secondly, if you won't inform the DVLA then I'm afraid we will have to. It's my duty to do so.'

I do like to lay the pomposity on when the opportunity arises.

Mr Bates stood up quickly, knocking his chair over in the process. 'You can't bloody snitch on me!' he shouted. 'You're my bleeding doctor, not a bleeding policeman! I ain't giving up my car!'

I persuaded him to sit back down so that I could arrange the necessary referral to confirm my diagnosis. But when he left a few minutes later, he was still muttering darkly.

After the door slammed behind Mr Bates, Lucie looked at me wide-eyed. 'My goodness,' she said. 'Is that sort of behaviour common? What happens next?'

'Sadly, it is common,' I said. 'And what happens next is I contact the DVLA, and hopefully, he complains about me.'

'*Hopefully*?' she said.

'There's no better feeling than receiving a letter of complaint when you know that you are absolutely and incontrovertibly in the right, Lucie.'

Bolshy patients resembling buses, the next one in was similarly stroppy.

She was Mrs Stagg, and she was demanding antibiotics for the snotty-nosed young daughter she'd brought with her. The trouble was, the child had nothing more serious than a common cold. Antibiotics attack bacterial infections, and colds are caused by viruses; antibiotics are to viruses what custard pies are to the Taliban.

I've never seen such a performance: I must have told her four times that the kid didn't need them, as Mrs Stagg became ever more agitated and Lucie's jaw dropped lower and lower. Finally, Mrs Stagg played her trump card. 'Look,' she said. 'I'm a veterinary nurse, so I know all about antibiotics. You don't need to patronise me. Are you saying I have to wait until my daughter gets sick and then take her to casualty to get what she needs?'

'No,' I said. 'How could you possibly say that? Your daughter doesn't *need* antibiotics. They will do her no good and they may even do her some harm. Therefore, they are a poison. I am a doctor. I don't poison children. Poisoning children is *not* my job. You will get exactly the same response at casualty, if the doctor there has any backbone.'

'But last time she got better.'

'Ah!' I said. 'Of course she did. But it doesn't mean... look, *post hoc ergo propter hoc.*'

'Eh?'

'It's Latin for "*after* this, therefore *because* of this". It's a logical fallacy. Your kid got better last time, but it was a coincidence, not because of the treatment. She doesn't need antibiotics for a snotty nose, and she ain't getting them from me.'

Another satisfied customer.

'Do you think she'll complain, too?' said Lucie.

'With any luck,' I said. 'She'll stick a letter into Jane Carstone, who'll lovingly pour petrol on the troubled flames before it all eventually goes away. By the time you get to my age, you perversely enjoy these conversations. If everything goes swimmingly for a week, you start to think, "Hang on, I'm losing my touch here... I should be disagreeing with the punters more. Am I just getting soft, and saying yes to everything?" There are times, understandably, when people want things they don't need. Sometimes it would just be a waste of money, but sometimes it can be downright dangerous. A big part of our job is to protect patients from themselves.'

MRS STAGG ISN'T THE ONLY ONE

THERE ARE A FEW things that everybody, not just Mrs Stagg, knows about antibiotics.

You can't drink if you're taking them.

Even if you don't need them for a sore throat, you do need them for sinusitis.

If you are prescribed them you must complete the whole seven day course.

Wrong, wrong and wrong again.

Patients try all sorts of tricks to get their hands on them, doctors play all sort of games in our efforts to restrict their use to situations where they might actually do more good than harm. The battle has been raging ever since Alexander Fleming discovered penicillin.

No-one ever tells me that they have a 'sore throat' any more, because they've seen all those posters saying 'Antibiotics Don't Work for Sore Throats'. Instead, they claim they have 'tonsillitis'. Tonsillitis, to a doctor, means 'sore throat'. Tonsillitis to a patient means 'sore throat that won't get better without penicillin'. *So hand it over*.

Similarly, hardly anyone now tells me that they've got a cough, a cold or the flu – not since the NHS produced all those posters saying that 'Antibiotics Don't Work for Coughs and Colds'. They tell me that they've got a 'chest infection', which is actually a completely meaningless term. The vast majority of respiratory infections are caused by viruses. Even the odd one or two that are caused by bacteria will probably get better just as quickly without antibiotics, assuming that the patient is otherwise well. We know this because we've done experiments with sugar pills and other subterfuges.

Aha! You might point out that patients who get pills of any kind (sugary or genuinely bactericidal) get better more quickly than patients who don't get anything but a gentle shove towards the exit. True, but if you want to be treated with placebos, go to a homoeopath. At least their sugar tablets aren't harmful; the antibiotics I use all have potential side effects.

Advanced players ring me on Monday morning, tell me that they came down with one of their attacks of sinusitis over the weekend but – and this is where I am supposed to feel grateful – they didn't bother me on Saturday morning because they had some left-over antibiotics from their last attack in their bathroom cabinet. So they started to take them and now all they need is a prescription for a few more to complete the course.

Of course, if I say no, this means that they can't take a whole week's worth, and then the antibiotics they've necked so far will just kill off the weedy germs, leaving the big ugly brutish bacteria behind who will then have lots of bug nookie, double their population every 20 minutes and cause frightful complications, which will eventually result in my patient's tragic and premature death, a Coroner's inquest and my name all over the front page of the local papers (again).

Except that – and I really don't think I should be telling you this, it's like a magician giving away the secrets of the 'sawing a girl in half' trick – this isn't the case. A couple of years ago, a bunch of boffins in Amsterdam found that patients who stopped taking their antibiotics when they felt better, even if that was before the end of the course, came to no harm.

There are two reasons why GPs don't normally tell their patients this.

Firstly, if you don't take all your tablets then you'll have a cache of unfinished packets of antibiotics in your bathroom cabinet so that you can play doctor or pull the Monday morning stunt in future.

Secondly... well, picture this. At the end of a 10 minute skirmish with a patient who absolutely demands a course of completely unnecessary antibiotics, my options are very limited – I can push the button that opens the trapdoor beneath the patient's chair to the shark-infested pool below my surgery, I can challenge the patient to a brief and violent exchange of views in the car park or I can issue a prescription designed to get them out of my room so I can get on with my work.

As Option One is still very much in the design and planning stage and Option Two is rarely if ever productive then that leaves me with Option Three – the Totally Spurious Prescription.

Human nature being what it is, after enduring 10 minutes' non-stop belittling of my diagnostic skills, my ethical imperative ('Above all, do no harm' and all that), my working knowledge of pathology and therapeutics and mainly because I am by now really, really pissed off, rest assured the antibiotic prescription that's whirring out of the printer is not one designed to minimise unwanted and unpleasant side effects.

It's a prescription that, although possibly justifiable on the very slimmest of medical grounds – that the patient's apparently trivial infection is not caused by a commonly occurring virus but by an unbelievably unlikely combination of potentially deadly bacteria – is virtually guaranteed to produce mouth ulcers, stomach cramps, nausea, explosive diarrhoea, an itchy rash (if I'm lucky) and a particularly unpleasant yeast infection involving the genitals.

And *that's* why I'll insist that he or she completes the whole seven day course.

CT SCANS

I NOTICED SOME INTERESTING developments on the graffiti front yesterday.

To the right of the door, all in the same silver pen:

> *KYLE CHUZLEWIT IS BENT MAN!*
> *Chuzlewit u r gay u no it*
> *Kyle Chuzlewit is sooooo g*

I stood for a moment, reflecting on the abrupt conclusion of the final sentence – interrupted, I imagined, by the connection of Kyle Chuzzlewit's fist with the author's head. It must have come as something of a shock.

Coincidentally, Mr Rouncewell came in later, complaining of headaches.

'They've been going on for a fortnight or so now, doctor,' he said. 'I've been taking paracetamol but they're not having much effect. I reckon I need a CAT scan.'

'I don't think that's a very good idea just yet,' I said. 'Do you know what a CT scanner is?'

'It's like a tube you lie in and they can look inside your head and see what the problem is,' he said. 'A bit like on *Star Trek*.'

'What it actually does is bombard you with multiple x-rays, giving a better and more detailed picture than a single x-ray. Computed tomography, it's called, hence "CT" or "CAT". A brilliant invention. British, actually – the Beatles essentially funded its development through their record sales, bizarrely. But that's not the whole story.'

'No?'

'No. You know that x-rays are dangerous, right?'

'Are they?'

'They are. They're radioactive, and exposure to radiation can cause cancer. That's why when you have one, the technician leaves the room and that buzzer sounds.'

'I always wondered why that was,' said Mr Rouncewell.

'X-rays are pretty safe, and the danger is generally outweighed by the benefits. If you've got a broken leg, we need to see the state the bone is in, and it's worth taking the tiny risk from the x-ray itself. But CT scans are like lots of x-rays at once – hundreds of them. I was reading recently about an American study which suggests that where people are CT-scanned as part of an asymptomatic screening programme – that's where the doctor sends you for a scan as part of a general check-up, just to see if there's anything wrong with you – they produce a net disbenefit. That is to say, they cause more new cancers than they actually find existing ones. It's beautifully ironic. Still, it's only Americans!'

'Right.'

'Then there's the anxiety factor,' I said, picking up my sphygmomanometer and gesturing to him to roll up his sleeve. 'Have you ever heard of an incidentaloma?'

'No.'

'The better CT and MRI scans get, the more we're realising that there's no such thing as normal. In fact, the only person who's normal is the person who hasn't been investigated hard enough. If you have your head CT-scanned, there's about a 5% chance that they *will* find something abnormal. But "abnormal" does not mean "problematic". It just means unusual. We call these things "incidentalomas" because they are entirely incidental to your health. There's no clinical issue, you'll have whatever it is your whole life and never know about it and die aged 90 with a Brazilian lingerie model in your arms. But if we pick it up on a scan… oooh, it freaks you out, you don't trust me when I say it's nothing, you want something done about it, and then it's brain biopsy time. That is the removal of a small piece of your actual brain tissue so some boffin with thick glasses in a lab somewhere can stick it under a microscope and come back and tell us what we already know, that it's nothing to worry about. By which time you've had your head cut open and you feel a lot, lot worse than you did when we started this conversation.'

I started taking his blood pressure.

'So what are you saying, doc?'

'I'm saying that there are a hundred possible explanations for your headache, and we don't need to go straight to the square marked "CT scan". You're worried that it's a brain tumour or high blood pressure, but tumours are vanishingly rare and your blood pressure's fine and doesn't really cause headaches anyway, so it's most likely caused by tension – the contraction of the muscles in your head and neck. That in turn can be caused by lots of things – stress, tiredness, boozing too much, sitting badly, eye strain – and fretting that you need a CT scan. Have you changed anything in the last couple of weeks?'

'I got a new job in a call centre.'

'Does it involve slobbing in front of a computer all day?'

'Well… yes.'

'On your way out, pop by reception and ask for one of their leaflets about posture and using a PC. Sit up straight, take screen breaks, have the monitor at eye level, that sort of thing. Meanwhile, try some ibuprofen as well as the paracetamol, and if things aren't better in a couple of weeks, come back and see me.'

'Is that *it*?' he said.

I could sense the disappointment in his voice. The thing lay people – and I include most politicians and medical academics in this, which is why protocols, guidelines and 'care pathways' are often bonkers – don't seem to understand about GPs is that, with most things we see, we don't *know* what's wrong at first, it's almost always too early in their evolution to be certain. So we often don't make diagnoses, we make *hypotheses* – it's probably A, but if X, Y or Z happens it's B, and then you should come back and see me. Hand on heart, I can't be absolutely sure that Mr Rouncewell *doesn't* have a brain tumour. I'm obviously not going to tell him that, but, for the reasons explained above, I equally can't send him for an immediate CT scan. If I did that with everyone who came through my door with a headache, the scanner would be working 24/7, we'd be causing hundreds of unnecessary deaths every year and the few poor sods who really *did* need scans would have to wait so long that they'd get an appointment with the undertaker first. So we proceed slowly, treating the most likely causes and assessing the response.

'I think so, for now,' I said. 'Maybe one day we'll have some sort of *Star Trek* wand I can wave over you to work out exactly what the problem is, but sadly this is 2010, not Stardate 1313.8. For now, as I was saying to a junior colleague just the other day, a big part of my job is to protect you from yourself.'

MORE ON SCANS

IF ALL THAT doesn't convince you, try this.

Fans of the excellent sitcom *Early Doors* will remember the episode where Duffy realises that the spark is going out of the relationship with his girlfriend. After a stolen afternoon of passion, he confesses to his mate that, even though his lover had worn her sexiest kit for a private and intimate photo-shoot, he hadn't even bothered to put any film in the camera.

Hold that thought.

Radiologist Dr Otto Chan, giving evidence at an employment tribunal, said that while working at the Royal London Hospital in 2006 he had found 100,000 unprocessed X-rays hidden in a cupboard.

One. Hundred. Thousand.

This proves my point: that some investigations are ordered because the doctor hopes to glean useful information from them, some are ordered as part of a routine and a great many are ordered simply to get the patient to vacate the consulting room chair to allow the next punter to sit down.

And it's these unnecessary investigations that cause so much trouble. Patients who win a consolation prize Full Blood Count, Chem Seven[1] and chest film by spending nine minutes describing symptoms that suggest pathology affecting every physiological process in the body are the *very* patients who will insist that their marginally-raised lymphocyte[2] count and borderline cardio-thoracic ratio[3] are investigated further. And further. And further. To no avail and at our expense. (By 'our', I mean 'your'.)

I'm starting a campaign for an extra tick box on the X-Ray request form: 'NTR NAD' – '*No Test Required, just supply report reading Nothing Abnormal Detected*'.

We would then use these for the many occasions when the dangers of a miniscule radiation dose would outweigh the investigation's negligible benefit.

---

[1] Testing the levels of blood urea, serum chloride, carbon dioxide, creatinine, blood glucose, serum potassium and serum sodium in the blood.

[2] Lymphocytes are white blood cells in the immune system: raised levels suggest viral infections or sometimes more serious problems.

[3] Put (very) simply, this describes the ratio between the size of the heart and of the chest. A larger than normal cardiothoracic ratio can point to heart failure and other issues.

REBECCA BAGNET AGAIN (AGAIN)

'YEAH, THANKS FOR ringing. And thanks again for helping us out.'

I was duty doctor, and I was fielding a phone call from the pharmacist at our local superstore.

The Senior Partner had given a patient a prescription for something to take the edge off her cervical spondylosis. In an effort to reduce the shooting pains down her arm, he'd tried a nerve-blocking drug called gabapentin; for the SP, this is messing with very modern medicines indeed, considering that he's only just given up on barbiturates and leeches.

I'm certain that he would have outlined the fairly complicated dosage instructions to her in the plainest English (take one tablet on the first day, one tablet every twelve hours on day two, one tablet every eight hours on day three, and then increase the dose according to response by adding in an additional tablet to the morning, afternoon and bedtime doses in turn to a maximum of four tablets per dose) but by the time she'd got to the chemist to have the prescription made up she'd forgotten everything.

The problem was that rather than type out the dosage instructions onto the prescription system to be printed out, the SP had simply labelled it to be taken 'as directed'.

Thank God you're here, Captain Chemist! My Hero! Not only did he get to make a 'Sorry to trouble you but I'm a smug pharmacist about to point out a prescribing error' phone call, he also got to label the process a 'Medicines Use Review' and claim a £25 bounty from the PCT. But still, I was genuinely grateful for his assistance.

'While I'm on,' he said. 'Did you know that the Bagnet family had moved house?'

'Huh?'

'You know, Matthew, Claire and Rebecca, the diabetic kid? I've just had a prescription from the Summerson Practice across town. A fortnight's supply of Lantus and Humalog for Becca, with an address in Jarndyce Drive.'

Hmmmm.

CHASING REBECCA

ON THE WAY back to Bleak House for the afternoon's Well Baby Clinic, I called the Summerson practice's by-pass number. A moment or two later I was chatting to Esther Summerson, local GP training supervisor and all round good egg.

'Just wondered if you remembered seeing a teenaged diabetic girl called Rebecca yesterday,' I said. 'She gave an address in Jarndyce but unless she's left home in a huff I've still got her living with her parents over my end of town.'

'Yeah,' said Esther. 'Goth girl? Thin as a rake? Came in as a Temporary Resident saying she'd left her insulin at home, so I gave her a couple of week's worth to tide her over. Have I screwed up?'

'No. Absolutely not. Thanks for doing it. I guess she was staying at her boyfriend's gaff.'

'Tony?'

'Yes?'

'Assuming she comes back to you, have a look at her teeth. I know she's a type 1 and all that, and that might explain the stick insect appearance, but painfully thin girl with bad teeth equals possible eating disorder. As she was only a TR I didn't think I should get involved. But.'

'Yeah, *but*. Thanks. I may well owe you one.'

PHARMACISTS

I FOUND MYSELF standing in a queue with all the other punters in a pharmacy yesterday.

Mrs Copperfield's mum was staying with us for the weekend. She's prone to coughs and wheezes, and for some reason she swears by Fisherman's Friends as a prophylactic. While I naturally don't much like queuing in a chemist's, I absolutely hate sitting listening to Mrs Copperfield's mum jabbering on, so at the first sight of a hanky I was up and out of the door on the hunt for a bag of those horrible northern lozenges.

Three hours later, I was standing in line, looking at the shelves of weird hair dyes and bottles of vitamin pills, idly wondering how long I could reasonably stretch this out for, when I overheard the young woman in front of me talking to the pharmacist.

Their conversation went like this:

Customer: 'I'm a contact lens wearer and I have sore eyes.'

Pharmacist (takes pack from shelf): 'I can't give you any drops. But you can use ibuprofen tablets.'

Customer: 'They'll help ease the pain, will they?'

Pharmacist: 'Yes. You could also do with something to boost your immune system. I'd suggest Echinacea.' Walks off to get some from elsewhere in shop, then pauses on his return. 'Come to think of it, you might as well take advantage of our 3-for-2 offer.'

Customer: 'Yes, anything that will help.'

Pharmacist: 'OK, I'd suggest these Vitamin C tablets.'

The pharmacist was incredibly polite and obliging. The patient was incredibly grateful. I, meanwhile, was just incredulous.

There was no mention of seeing an optician or a GP, and you don't need 10 years at med school to know that undiagnosed ocular problems should not be treated with one painkiller and two placebos – especially in contact lens wearers, who can suffer some particularly nasty eye infections.

I probably should have intervened, but I was so stunned that by the time I gathered my wits the woman had left the shop.

Shocking as it was, it was all of a piece with the general drift towards the idea that you don't really need to consult a doctor about your problems if you can get hold of a bloke in a white coat behind a counter in the High Street – a bloke, by the way, who *won't* send you to me when he should (see above) but who *will* when he shouldn't (hint: snot is supposed to be green – don't direct patients to me for antibiotics when they actually just need a pack of tissues).

I shuffled forwards and picked up a packet of Fisherman's Friends, still slightly disbelieving.

'That'll be 70p please,' said the pharmacist.

As I fished in my pocket for the coins, my eye ranged across the shelves of placebos – sorry, cough mixtures, vitamins and tonics – arrayed before me.

Look, I know I shouldn't be having a go at the chemists, and that we should be running hand-in-hand through soft focus fields of corn in a combined and harmonious primary care effort to save our patients from the evils of dry skin, warts and rhinoviruses. But the point is this. In modern medicine, pharmacists are being promised a much bigger role. Fine. I've no doubt they're bright enough and keen enough. But I do have reservations about sharing my patients and my workload with people who on the one hand want to be serious medical professionals and on the other want to run a shop, because those two roles don't sit comfortably together. If pharmacists could decide amongst themselves whether they want to sell cough drops or become quasi-doctors then maybe we could make some progress.

THE SUSPICIONS OF MR NICKLEBY

'I'VE STILL GOT that buzzing in my ear.'

Huh? Hang on. Do I know anything about this? He marched in, plonked himself down and just started talking.

'That buzzing? I've still got it.'

And quite a lot more, as he went on to tell me.

I scanned his notes. *Mr Nickleby*. I'd never laid eyes on him before. He'd shopped around everyone else with his polysymptomatic litany of despair, but no-one had ever found anything wrong with him, despite multiple tests. And no-one had seemed able to help him, despite a variety of 'therapeutic trials'.

Many symptoms + frequent attendance + zero success = a ghastly feeling whenever a bloke like this walks into the room.

In other words, Mr Nickleby is a gold plated, copper bottomed, cast iron heartsink.

After a perfunctory chat and an even briefer examination, I cut to the chase. What this man needed was a dose of 'continuity of care'. But not from me. I've got enough on my plate, thanks.

'The thing is,' I said, 'When someone has... er... *complex* problems like yours, it's really important to stick with one doctor.'

'Well, I'll stick with you, then,' he said.

I pretended not to hear this. 'And I see your usual doctor is Dr Patel, so you really should book an appointment...'

'Nah, I'd rather stick with you.'

I tried another tack. 'But it might be worth you seeing our very experienced senior partner – he has a particular interest in ear, nose and throat problems...'

'Nah, I've decided I'll stick with you.'

'…or our registrar, Dr Lucie, a young, up-to-date doctor who I'm sure could shed new light on…'

'No, really, I'll stick with you.'

Oh, sod it.

'It's worse when I lean to one side.'

'What is?'

'That buzzing in my ear.'

HEARTSINKS

I MENTIONED THAT Mr Nickleby was a 'heartsink'. The term is derived from that feeling a GP gets when he sees a given patient's name on the appointment list yet again. You might think it is pejorative, and perhaps it is (a little), but it's still a whole lot better than its predecessor, 'Hateful Patients'; and it does sum up the feeling of dread and the 'here we go again' sensation that the very mention of particular person's name can conjure up in his doctor.

They tend to be women (fact, not prejudice) from lower social classes (ditto) and in the days when we wrote notes on bits of paper they would have huge 'fat files' – brimming over with out-patient clinic letters, test results and records of their (incredibly) frequent GP appointments.

(I know one doctor with a patient who has clocked up 1,500 appointments in the last ten years, or an average of three visits a week *every* week. If we had a patient like that we'd change the locks, but we certainly have some who come in once a week on average.)

As a rule, heartsinks tend to book a ten minute appointment but expect to be seen for twenty, and they seem to take perverse pleasure in telling their doctor that the last treatment they were given didn't work (just like the one before, and the one before that).

They insist on trying the latest miracle cure they read about in *Take A Break* or heard about on daytime TV, even when it's patently inappropriate, and constantly ask for second (and third and even fourth) opinions, as well as pointless investigations.

Each GP has, on average, a dozen to cope with on his list of patients at any one time. In a particularly tough morning surgery he may well encounter all of the Big Four.

1. *The Entitled Demander*. This patient really doesn't like GPs (or hospital docs who fail to supply a miracle cure or small print diagnoses). He thinks of me as an obstacle to get around to secure more tests and treatments – and he's probably right. In his case, that's my job.

2. *The Dependent Clinger*. These folks appear grateful for the help they're getting, but bombard me with symptom after symptom after symptom (after symptom after symptom after symptom) and expect me to reassure them, even if to do so would be inappropriate. The symptoms they describe hardly ever fit in to any recognisable pattern of illness, and when they do it's bastard difficult to put the jigsaw pieces in the right place while being peppered with other pieces from other puzzles.

3. *The Manipulative Help-rejecter* is the lady who loves to tell me how badly I'm doing. When I suggest something that might be helpful, like losing weight (she'd have to start smoking again to do that) trying some tablets (but they never agree with her) or taking up a gentle exercise program (with *her* feet? I must be joking), she has the answer lined up. The only people who suffer more at her hands than I do are her family, who she twists around her little finger.

4. Finally, there are *The Self-destructive Deniers*. Uniquely among the heartsink fraternity, these patients are usually, and often quite seriously, ill. What makes them impossible to deal with is their complete inability to accept that their own actions might be adversely affecting their health – like the alcoholic who won't stop drinking even though his liver is shot.

One caveat to all of this: it has been argued that there are no heartsink patients, only heartsink doctors – in other words the issue is not with the patient but with me, because I don't have the nous to deal with the complex problems these patients present. But that's bollocks, obviously.

MANAGERS AND POLITICIANS

I SPENT THE morning with Henry Gowan, our incumbent medical student.

Unlike Lucie Manette, who is a registrar in her final year of training, Henry is just on attachment from med school for a few weeks. We get them in every now and then – they sit in on surgeries, do projects, make coffee etc and may even get to see a few patients on their own (we check up later to make sure they don't kill *too* many people). We've had Henry for the last week or so. He's very posh: his dad is some legal bigwig, he drives a car worth three times more than mine and he looks like Martin Fry out of ABC. He talks like a trustafarian gangsta, and naturally he and Sami bonded on sight.

Despite all that, he's not a bad lad.

After a morning of vomiting toddlers, incontinent old folks and constipated heartsinks we grabbed half an hour for lunch in the common room.

I suppose I ought to have spent the time chatting through the 'issues' 'raised' by the day's consultations, but the only issues they had really raised – in my mind, at least – were:

1) How long have I got till retirement?

and

2) Where are the Hob Nobs? (I hope you're spotting this product placement McVitie's.)

Henry started playing with his iPod or meFone or whatever, and I picked up a copy of *Pulse*, the excellent trade mag for GPs. (I would say this, since I am a columnist for the magazine.)

Five seconds later, I spat coffee all over it. Henry looked over, a laconic eyebrow raised.

'One of the joys of general practice,' I said, wiping biscuit crumbs off my shirt and waving the *Pulse* at him, 'is that you never quite know what's going to happen next.'

'Yeah, I feel you, man,' said Henry, by way of agreement. 'It's like… check it, yeah? When a patient walks through that door, it could be, like, absolutely anything, and you're expected to, like, deal with it?'

Why must everybody under 25 end every sentence with this ridiculous upwards inflection?

'No, that's not quite what I meant,' I said. 'When a patient walks through the bloody door, 99% of the time I know *exactly* what it's going to be… a plea for antibiotics, a sick note or a housing letter.'

And *they* know that the answer is, invariably, bugger off, bugger off and bugger off, so why do they bother? But that's another tutorial.

'No, I'm talking about the way managers and politicians keep messing around with primary care in different but ever-more ludicrous ways.'

Across the room, the Senior Partner looked up from his *Times*. 'What are they doing now?' he said.

'It says here that NHS managers in London are planning to reduce the length of GP consultations by a third,' I said. 'Apparently, some time and motion clowns reckon the NHS can make efficiency savings by closing hospitals, cancelling follow-ups and shifting a huge volume of work to primary care.'

The Senior Partner snorted. 'Clowns alright,' he said. 'I wonder if they asked any GPs what they thought? Or just stuck their fingers in the air to see which way the wind was blowing? I should have gone into bloody management consultancy.'

'Apparently, NHS London has refused Freedom of Information Act requests to release the report,' I said. 'Well, there's a surprise.'

'Why do they want to reduce appointment lengths?' said Henry. 'Am I, like, missing something?'

'Just a bit,' I said. 'If they're going to cut A&E attendance by 60% and outpatient appointments by 55% and put more of that work our way, there are three ways they can do it. They can quadruple the number of GPs, or they can create a 52-hour working day, or they can try putting a pint-and-a-half into a pint pot. Since the first is impractical on the grounds that the country is broke and the latter two are impossible due to the laws of physics, they are going to have to expand the size of the pint pot... er... they need to minimise the size of the... look, they need to get the GPs to see more patients per day.'

'OK,' said Henry. 'Fair point. But is that such a bad thing?'

'That *was* you sitting next to me this morning while I dealt with Mrs Mowcher's tired-all-the-time-with-a-bad-back-and-a-touch-of-dizziness-and-while-I'm-here-I've-got-this-patch-of-dry-skin, was it? And Mr Wardle's swollen-knee-with-headaches-and-weird-flashing-lights-and-possible-veruca-with-a-hint-of-breathlessness?

Because, if it was, and you think I can deal with people like that – which is pretty much *all* our people – in 10 minutes, never mind six minutes and 40 seconds, I'm all ears, Henry. The reality is, by the time I've done the meeting and greeting, fed the QOF monster and said, "What can I do for you today?", time will be up.'

With the result that, for this strain, that fed-up feeling and the other slight twinge in the chest I'll be sending punters to A&E, dishing out antidepressants and referring to Outpatients, respectively. Which, given that the agenda is to save money, kind of defeats the object. In fact, taking this strategy to its logical conclusion, future interactions will last less than a minute.

'Eventually we'll be expected to have finished the consultation before it's started,' I said.

'Before the patient's even booked the appointment, more like,' said the Senior Partner. 'All this in a system allegedly devoted to quality and patient choice and evidence-based medicine. How the hell are you supposed to listen effectively and have half a chance of diagnosing, or even hypothesising, under that kind of time pressure?'

'My brother works in management consultancy,' said Henry. 'He earns a bloody fortune.'

'Is he a clown?' I said, but he was miles away.

'I might see if they have any vacancies,' he said.

MR NICKLEBY RIDES AGAIN

'I'VE STILL GOT that buzzing in my ear.'

Ah. Mr Nickleby. Of course. He's back. And this time it's serious.

'I don't come very often, so I've brought a list.'

Deep joy. My knuckles are already white.

Rule One of 'Managing patients with lists', as I explained to Lucie Manette in a tutorial the other day, is, *get control of the list*.

So I did.

'Let's have a look at that, shall we? Hmmm. Buzzing in the ears… well, I think we knew that… tiredness… dizziness… not sleeping well… off your food…'

Rule Two of lists: Step back, take an overview and see if, against the odds, all those symptoms might *actually* add up to something, anything.

If not, go to Rule Three: Allow the patient to perm any three from the fifteen.

'I wonder if you might be depressed, Mr Nickleby?'

He looked affronted. 'Of course I'm bloody depressed,' he said. 'So would you be, with all those symptoms. There's more on the back.'

I turned the paper over. So there was. 'Headaches… spots in the eyes… a rash… creaking knees…'

'Have you been passing clumps of hair in your urine?' I said.

He looked startled. 'No? Why?'

'Oh, no reason,' I said. 'Something obscure I always keep my eye out for. Since you seem to have almost everything else, I wondered if…'

'No,' he said. 'Sorry.'

By then, I'd had my fun and so had he. I moved onto Rule Four of lists: Bin it.

Before he could protest, I whipped out a blood test form.

'We'd better check this out,' I said, filling in his details, and pausing for quite a while as I wondered what to write in the 'clinical problem' section. 'There. Take that to reception and book an appointment for a couple of weeks, when we should have the results.'

And when I shall be on holiday.

SEX MANIACS

THE FIRST PATIENT I saw last Tuesday was a 58-year-old forklift truck driver with skirt on his mind.

'I need some of that Viagra, doc,' said Mr Leeford, with admirable candour. 'The missus wants a bit more of the old how's-your-father than I can supply these days, if you know what I mean.'

For a moment, my mind drifted back to the good old sepia-tinged days of, ooh, nine or ten years ago.

Back 'in the day', we used to have what we called the 'hand-on-knob' consultation. Some chap would come in complaining that he had an ingrowing toenail, I would spend the allotted ten minutes looking at the healthiest set of feet in the county and, as he was leaving, he would pause, hand on the doorknob and an expression of anguished embarrassment about his *mien*.

'And? Is there anything else?' I'd say, my voice tinged with impatience.

'Er,' he'd say, hesitantly. 'Well…' And then he would pluck up the courage to point tentatively pantwards and say: 'Just before I go, can you help me out with a little problem I have… downstairs?'

Trust me, the frustration these impotent men felt was nothing compared with mine. With a heaving waiting room outside, I'd often cut to the chase after 30 seconds of the 'I've come about my cold, doctor' routine: 'Look, you haven't got nasal catarrh at all, have you?' I'd say. 'Come on, out with it – you're impotent, aren't you?'

On the upside, after a while I began to see very few men with nasal catarrh.

On the downside, there wasn't much we could do about the real problem.

There was psychosexual counselling, of course, but to the average bloke that is about as enjoyable as sticking needles in your penis. And then there was *actually* sticking needles in your penis and... well, would you?

All that changed with the arrival of Viagra. It works, it's painless and it's even trendy – and that, together with the rebadging of impotence to 'erectile dysfunction', has allowed Mr Floppy to stride out of the closet with a confident air and his hand outstretched. Some days, I have as much trouble keeping up as the patients do.

That said, I don't dish out the magic pills willy-nilly, as it were.

'The thing about Viagra, Mr Leeford,' I said, 'is that it's strictly rationed.'

'Rationed?'

'Yes. Most men have to pay for it. There are a few who get it on the NHS – men with diabetes, or MS, or post-prostate cancer surgery, one or two other categories – but even they don't get more than four tablets per month.'

'Four tablets a month! I'd need four a night to keep up with her!'

'It's the Dobson Ration, you see.'

'The Dobson Ration?'

'Yes, Frank Dobson. Beardy fellow, slightly fat. Some people thought he was a bit simple, though it's not for me to say. He was the Health Secretary when Viagra came in, and he decided that one amorous encounter a week was quite enough for anyone, for which I imagine Mrs Dobson was eternally grateful. If you do qualify under the NHS – and you don't – then you pay the normal prescription charge. Otherwise it's a private prescription. Including the dispensing fee, that's £62.50 for eight 100mg tablets, I'm afraid.'

He sat back in his chair, the wind gone from his sails. 'But that's bloody outrageous,' he said. 'This problem only started when that Dr Emma gave my missus the bloody HGV.'

'Do you mean HRT?'

'Yeah, that's the one. She's a changed woman ever since. It's killing me, I tell you.'

'Well, I sympathise – not from any position of personal experience, you understand – but you don't tick any of the necessary boxes so there's not a great deal I can do for you, Viagra-wise.'

I wrote him a private prescription, and he left looking rather crestfallen, with a slightly hunted expression in his eyes. Clearly, the tigerish Mrs Leeford was waiting for him back at base.

FAKING IT

THAT LUNCHTIME, OVER a supermarket chicken salad sarnie which cost £3 and tasted mostly of cardboard, I got chatting to Sami Patel about Viagra.

'I reckon most blokes I turn down for an NHS script just go home, open the spam folder in their email inbox and send off for some fakes,' he said.

'You're probably right,' I said.

'Of course I'm right. Think about it. You can buy generic 100mg sildenafil tablets made in India and China for about £2 apiece on the internet, so who's going to pay the pharmacy rate? Ask yourself this, of all the guys you've ever prescribed an ED drug who don't qualify on the NHS, how many of them *ever* return for a repeat prescription? Have you ever bothered to ask why?'

He had a point. Our local pharmacist has recently adorned his window with a home-made, A4 poster warning passers-by, 'Don't buy drugs off the internet'.

What he doesn't mention is that of the sixty quid your eight Viagra tablets will cost you, a third of that is his 'dispensing fee'. Nice work if you can get it: £23 to take a packet down off a shelf and stick a label on it.

Of course, the pharmacy industry's spokesmen talk more about the dangers of shopping for meds online: they'd have you believe that every product supplied is counterfeit, cut with toilet cleaner and a danger to health. And, to be fair, one in four GPs reckons he or she has treated a patient who has suffered a side effect from a drug bought online without a prescription. But when you consider that *four* out of four of us have treated patients suffering side effects of drugs we've actually prescribed ourselves, you might argue those aren't bad odds.

Obviously, I'm no more going to advise you to buy your 'Propecia' or 'Prozac' online than I'd suggest you buy the brake pads for your car from a back-street set-up in Mumbai. 'Original parts' for my 'Nissam' or 'Toyata'? Er, na thonks (and I'm not being ironic here, I really mean this – *don't* buy pills off the internet). But we live in the real world, and most patients ignore everything I say anyway.

Fire up your web browser and Google any of the generic names for P5 inhibitors (the chemical class of drugs that includes Viagra, Cialis and Levitra); within seconds you'll find links to Indian and Chinese manufacturers who knock out unlicensed generic product. These aren't always shifty blokes with buckets of powdered chalk and a printing press in a lock-up; they're often the same firms that manufacture the beta-blockers, antibiotics and anti-inflammatories that pharmacists hand out quite happily in exchange for an FP10.

Just then, Dr Emma came in.

'Ah!' I said. 'Just the girl I wanted to see.'

'Really?' she said. 'Has anyone seen my coffee mug?'

Sami shifted guiltily. 'Er, I think I used it earlier,' he said. 'It's in the sink.'

'You *think* you used it?' said Dr Emma. She walked to the sink. 'It's chipped!' she said. 'You've chipped my coffee mug! That was an original Greenpeace "Don't Make A Wave" mug. It cost me £25 on eBay!'

'Gosh, is that the time?' said Sami Patel. 'I really must…'

The rest was lost as he slid out of the common room.

'Shame about your mug, Emma,' I said. 'Look, can you do me a favour, and stop prescribing HRT to every slightly sweaty woman over 45 who darkens your door? It's causing mayhem with their menfolk.'

'I don't know what you mean,' she said. 'Don't be so ridiculous. I don't prescribe anything to anyone who doesn't need it.'

'Look,' I said. 'I know we don't dish out HRT like we used to, not since people started accepting the menopause as a natural part of the ageing process. But it's still a damn sight easier to get hold of than Viagra, thanks to the inherent sexism in the NHS.'

'Oh, you're not going to start banging on about that again, are you?' she said. 'It's a bit of a stuck record, Tony.'

'It's a fact, you mean,' I said. 'Look at the way we pour money into cervical and mammographic screening, which are exclusively female and, in diagnostic terms, clinically controversial. All this talk of women GPs for female patients, and never a murmur about a reciprocal arrangement for blokes. Free contraception for women, while men have to cough up for condoms. For years, HRT was handed out to pretty much any woman who asked. When Viagra arrived, a drug for blokes that was – for once – fashionable, it was immediately rationed. The fact is, men's health isn't politicised, and this whole Viagra/HRT thing is the clearest evidence of that.'

PIERCINGS, TATTS
AND OLD MEN WITH THE CLAP

ACTUALLY, IT WAS a day for sex maniacs of one sort or another.

On the way back to my consulting room, I bumped into another of them, in the slightly potato-shaped shape of the reception manager, Mrs Peggotty.

'Now then, Dr Copperfield?' she said, in her warm, Irish brogue. 'Can I just ask you, would you have had unprotected sex, or been pierced or tattooed lately?'

'That's rather forward, Mrs Peggotty,' I said. 'I mean, I had a big night last Friday but I certainly wouldn't…'

'No, you big silly,' she said, playfully slapping my arm. 'It's just this new poster which came today.'

She held it up; an horrific teenaged Goth stared back at me under a heading which asked about sex, piercings and tatts. I think it was designed to warn our local yoot as to the terrors of hepatitis B, the blood-borne variety of the virus, but I fear most of them will see it as more of an ad: a good percentage of them appear to regard all three activities as essential components of a good evening.

I walked through the waiting area and back to my desk.

My final patient of the day turned out to be precisely the sort of oddbod the poster was aimed at – though he was slightly older than you might have thought.

Mr Maylie, a middle-aged office manager with a gammy leg and a lazy eye, didn't waste any time in getting to the point.

'I think I've got a dose, doc,' he said, with a knowing wink. 'I used to be in the army in the '70s and I reckon I know the signs.'

A quick inspection revealed that he did, and he had.

'So you're enjoying an adventurous sex life, are you?' I said, struggling to keep the bitterness out of my voice.

'Well, there's Jackie in accounts, and Margaret at the Red Lion, and Smutty Sal from the cab firm, and…'

'I've heard enough,' I said. 'For God's sake, stop.'

I gave him a stern lecture as to the importance of morality – or, at least, condoms – and sent him on his way to the clap clinic so they could do the tests to find out exactly what type of VD he had.

It seems odd discussing safe sex with people of his age – who ought to be more worried about infarction than infection – but at least the conversation tends to go beyond, 'Whatever'. And it's becoming an increasingly important conversation to have. I don't know if you realise this, but the middle aged and even elderly are experiencing an epidemic of sexually-transmitted diseases – a 'clapidemic', I like to call it. A recent Health Protection Agency study showed that sexually-transmitted infections, such as genital warts, herpes and gonorrhoea, have doubled in the middle aged, particularly in men over 45, in the last decade or so.

Since the arrival of the aforementioned Viagra, the quickie divorce and the internet (sites like Friends Reunited have opened up lots of old doors from days gone by), people in their forties, fifties and above are enjoying bedroom action of the sort which was previously confined to the orgiasts of ancient Rome. (Or so I hear – it's not like that in my house, obviously.)

Add in the menopausal binning of condoms and you have a recipe for disaster. Well, unpleasant oozing and odd penile growths, anyway.

AIRFIX MAN

BY NOW, YOU may be drawing up a mental image of me as a burnt-out old cynic whose relationship with his patients is akin to that of a molar with a drill.

If so, you're almost completely right. Except that, occasionally, something like this happens.

Mr Haredale came to see me the other day.

He's 80 years old, and was sprightly, smiley and superbly turned-out. His attendance record is exemplary, in the sense that he hardly ever comes and he apologises for bothering us when he does.

As soon as he popped his head round the door, I recognised him and started putting the AK-47 – always primed for action at the beginning of any consultation – back in its drawer.

'I've just got the one problem, doctor,' he said, and I felt my default *froideur* melt still further. 'It's these shakes. By the time I get from the kitchen to my armchair, my tea's in the saucer. I've had them for ages and I'm about fed up with it.'

Typical essential tremor. He was a lovely man and this was a straightforward problem, so I turned Nice Family Doctor up to max.

'You're probably worried it's Parkinson's, aren't you Mr Haredale?' I said. 'Well, it isn't, so you can relax on that score.'

He exhaled deeply and sat back, a weight off his shoulders. 'Well, that's good to hear, doctor,' he said.

'But you say you've had it for ages, so why's it worrying you now?'

'It's my Airfix models,' he explained. 'I can't do the fiddly bits anymore. I've got a lovely 1:24 scale model of *HMS Hood* on the go and I just can't get the Oerlikons... they were the anti-aircraft guns... I just can't get them sited properly. I knew a chap who died on the

Hood, as it happens. Lovely lad. He was the butcher's son. They never got over it.'

He looked downwards at his shaky hands.

This is enough to get him to bother the GP?

Well, actually, yes, and rightly so. Because his wife died three years ago, and his hobby fills in those moments when he'd otherwise be pining for her, which is all the time.

My own hands used to tremble when I did Airfix kits, but that was because I was a six-year-old banished to the Arctic temperatures of the garden shed, so it wasn't just my hands shaking, it was my whole body. Maybe that was why Mr Haredale touched me so much. Or maybe it was just that this consultation cut through the dross and reminded me why I do this job. It may be a cliché that doctors need to have an interest in people as well as pathology, but it's a trait of all decent GPs, albeit one which gets buffeted and eroded by the moaning, manipulative, multisymptomatic masses.

The tiny minority who create the vast majority of our work distort our view and pervert our attitude. Most of humanity gets by each day without consulting, phoning or complaining, it's just that it doesn't always feel like that to us GPs. So maybe we should have an 'Infrequent Attenders Day', when we invite all Thin-Files for a consultation. Most wouldn't come, and those who did wouldn't bring lists or say 'While I'm here', so we could OD on caffeine and Hob Nobs.

Perfect.

As for Mr Haredale, I suggested he tries a little Glenmorangie. Then maybe we'll give beta-blockers a go. If we're still stuck, hell, I'll go round and do the fiddly bits for him myself.

PARKINSON'S DISEASE

UNLIKE MR HAREDALE, around 1 in 500 Britons – or 120,000 people in total – *do* have Parkinson's, with some 10,000 new cases diagnosed each year, mostly in patients over 50. Named after the London doctor James Parkinson who first identified it in 1817, it is a progressive neurological condition caused by the loss of nerve cells in a part of the brain called the substantia nigra, where dopamine is produced; this chemical helps the brain to co-ordinate movement and its depletion causes patients to struggle with walking, talking and other activities. It is 'idiopathic' in nature, which means that its causes are not yet fully understood; however, they are thought to include genetic factors and exposure to environmental toxins, herbicides and pesticides. There is no current cure, but there are treatments and therapies which can alleviate the symptoms.

Essential Tremor is a less serious condition which sees patients trembling involuntarily. Alcohol intake – in moderation, of course – can reduce the symptoms (which is why so many snooker and darts players have been boozers) and drugs including beta blockers, which work by blocking the transmission of certain nerve impulses, are also used.

THINGS I REALLY LIKE ABOUT GENERAL PRACTICE

I MENTIONED THAT Mr Haredale was superbly turned out.

Coming from me, who often turns up to work looking like a *Big Issue* seller, that might strike you as odd. But there's something about the sight of an old suit and a frayed shirt collar held together by a well-pressed tie that brings out the softy in me.

You may think my outlook on life, and particularly work, is relentlessly bleak, and that it is thus doing bugger all for recruitment. If so, it looks like I'm hitting the spot. But, to redress the balance, here's a list of all the things I really like about general practice.

Obviously, frail widowers who attend resplendent in tie and jacket (even if they put me to shame).

I also like elderly ladies who decline scripts for paracetamol or aspirin because they'll buy them instead, to save the NHS some money. That's excellent – if everyone took that attitude with the drug budget, the same old ladies would be able to get their hip replacements done in time for them to actually enjoy their new-found mobility.

I like child patients who talk to me. Most don't. Most cough, pout, whine, puke, wail, scream, or all of the above. Yesterday, I asked a boy with earache how old he was and he said, 'Five. But before that I was four.' Encouraged by this, I asked him why he'd come. Without hesitation, he replied, 'To play with your toys.' Brilliant.

What else? I like patients who bring me presents, even if I don't like the presents. I've tried hard to develop a fondness for Liebfraumilch and lardy cake but it's not possible.

Then there are relatives who offer me tea on a visit. Marvellous. I've never accepted, though: there's always the outside chance that they're trying to poison me. This would be understandable – half an hour previously I was suggesting to them on the phone that faecal incontinence and complete immobility in a 95-year-old shouldn't necessarily be seen as barriers to bringing the patient to the surgery.

I'm nearing the bottom of the barrel now. I do quite like it when patients say amusing things.

Such as, 'Doctor, I need counselling'. This doesn't sound that amusing but it is, because they usually want counselling on spurious grounds, such as Birmingham City being relegated.

Also, I like that feeling you get when the patient's body language indicates that he's about to leave. The pleasure of closure; the sense of progression towards coffee; the impression of your career clock ticking from consultation 143,999 to 144,000, with only another 153,000 to go. Yes, I have just worked that out, and, no, it probably isn't healthy. Sadly, in most of those 153,000 remaining consultations, there will be a list, a 'while I'm here', a TATT. Occasionally there will something nasty. Set against this monument of negativity, my reasons to be cheerful do look slightly flimsy. Which is why, if you want to know the truth, I'm more likely to be humming AC/DC's *Highway To Hell* than Julie Andrews' *Favourite Things* on the road in to work of a Monday. But, hey, if you're a registrar or a student reading this, don't let that put you off.

SURELY EVERYONE IN TOWN HASN'T GOT A URINARY TRACT INFECTION?

'HAVE YOU EVER noticed,' asked Sami Patel, as we walked to our cars, 'how everyone we send to the hospital turns out to have a urinary tract infection? In the last fortnight, off the top of my head, I've had patients attend A&E with heart attacks, broken ankles, tonsillitis and suspected rabies and every single one of them has turned out to have problems in the waterworks as well.'

'I have noticed that, Sami,' I said. 'And in fact, I can top-trump your little collection.'

And I told him a story. A true one. The other day, an elderly patient of mine called Mr Feeder suddenly went numb and weak all the way down one side. His wife, understandably alarmed by the flaccid and slobbery appearance of one half of her husband, took him up to the local hospital. I know all this because I've got the A&E letter in front of me.

It states: 'Diagnosis: TIA'

A transient ischaemic attack, or mini-stroke: even a Cas. Officer couldn't get that wrong.

Hang on, though. That's just diagnosis number one. There was another.

Diagnosis number two, according to the letter is, as you will have guessed, a 'UTI.'

So, as I said to Sami, 'You see what he had?'

Sami looked blank.

'No idea?' I said. 'I'll put you out of your misery. He had….a UTIA. Geddit?'

As medical jokes go, it was quite a good one. In fact, so proud was I of this mini-stroke of genius that I repeated it to the senior partner over coffee.

'It's appalling really,' I said. 'You'd think the casualty officers would know that dipsticking the urine of any ill person has a good chance of turning up something untoward.'

This is true; coincidental 'abnormalities' of no clinical significance are often found in urine when it is tested – particularly when the patient is ill. These abnormalities are often irrelevant in the great scheme of things. They can sometimes be a sign of a urinary infection, true, but more often they are misinterpreted as such by doctors who are either misinformed or are looking for something to blame symptoms on.

'But "something untoward" does not a UTI make,' I continued. 'What the hell do they teach them nowadays?'

I sat there trying to work out a 'Taking the piss' joke, but the SP interrupted my thoughts.

'Actually, Tony, it's you I'm surprised at,' he said. 'You're being so naïve. It's obvious what's going on.'

'It is?'

'Of course,' he said. 'It's gaming. The hospital can charge the PCT more when they see a patient and perform a test. So TIA equals one fee. TIA plus urinalysis equals a bigger fee. It generates maximum dosh from the one attendance. Plus, of course, there's bound to be something in the wee, as you say. So it gives the casualty doctor an excuse to stop thinking. Whatever the symptoms, he can blame it on a UTI.'

Blimey. I tend not to get involved in local medicopolitics. Words like 'commissioning' and 'business plan' bring me out in a cold sweat. Not because, as the patient's advocate, I'm supposed to rise above that kind of thing – it's just that understanding these words obliges you to sit on endless committees with people who use jargon of this type routinely rather than the English language and, frankly, life's too short.

So I don't know if this casualty dysfunction really is financial manipulation or just stupidity. On the basis that I don't believe you can a train casualty doctor to follow any sort of protocol, let alone one that screws the system, I'll opt for the latter. But given how the medical profession likes to play whatever game is imposed, I could well believe the former.

GRANNY STACKERS AND LOLINADS

I TURNED ON the radio on the way in to work this morning, hoping to catch the latest twist in the weird and ongoing saga of Portsmouth FC, the club I have the misfortune of following.

Instead, my ears were assaulted by Nicky Campbell informing me that lots of Lolinads aren't getting the medicines they need. (For the uninformed, Lolinads are Little Old Ladies In No Apparent Distress.)

Seven out of ten Lolinads were said to be the victims of drug errors picked up during a series of half day visits to an assortment of granny stackers (nursing and residential homes) by a bunch of Herberts with clipboards.

The report said nothing about the seriousness of the errors, but here's a clue: out of 178 'victims', only one was said to have suffered a significant consequence, which was described as a 'thyroid complication'. This means that his or her levothyroxine dose was a little bit too high or a little bit too low, which puts him or her in the same bracket as most of my patients, given that I only check their thyroid numbers once a year and their meds are daily.

Another interesting point is that the article upon which this edifice of angst was built appeared not in the *British Medical Journal* but in that rather less august publication, *Quality & Safety in Health Care*.

That didn't prevent Help The Concerned Aged from pouring out their shock and anger to Nicky.

I must confess, I was genuinely taken aback, too.

How is it possible to screw up on no less than 178 occasions and only harm one patient? And even then, only to inflict nothing more than a biochemical flesh wound?

OK, with my Health & Safety hard hat and goggles firmly on, giving Mrs Scroggins her paracetamol at 8am rather than 6am might be classed as a 'mistake'. So might giving her a dose of tetracycline twenty minutes away from milk or food rather than thirty, handing out her statin at 6pm rather than bedtime and not making sure that she sits bolt upright for at least half an hour after her weekly dose of aledronate.

But get real. The last course of medication I took (a three-month course of an antifungal drug called terbinafine for a manky toenail) would have thrown up a list of drug errors that would keep the researchers occupied for a week. I'd say I missed every sixth dose, on average, and took the other pills at whatever moment I remembered them with whatever liquid was near to hand, if any.

I didn't run a sequential series of liver function tests, on the grounds that the terbinafine couldn't do me much more harm than the Jack Daniels, gin and Draught Bass were already doing.

It took 14 weeks to complete the course rather than 12. So what?

I'm not pretending that mistakes don't happen. A local nursing home lost a patient on methotrexate (which is bone-marrow toxic) a couple of years ago because the GPs expected the nurses to know that three-monthly blood counts were *de rigeur* and the nurses expected the GPs to remind them. An audit showed that every other at-risk patient on the practice's books was being tested like clockwork.

But setting out to panic the nation's army of concerned relatives is not the way forward.

I switched off the radio as I pulled into the Senior Partner's parking space at the surgery. Graffiti-wise, one new line: '*Kyle Chuzzlewit rule this hood u no it*' was written on the glass panel next to the door. Since the PCT showed no sign of removing any of the unofficial adornments to Bleak House, I resolved to bring in a scouring pad and some bleach from home.

REBECCA BAGNET: MORE WARNING SIGNS

ANOTHER DAY, ANOTHER steaming pile of incoming mail.

'Dr Copperfield, have you heard the latest news about the treatment of restless legs?'

Nope. Shred.

'Dear Doctor, how many of your patients are suffering from troublesome foot and ankle disorders?'

No idea. Shred.

'Dear Dr Copperfield, I'm afraid I really can't afford to waste any more of my appointment slots on this young lady. If and when the time comes when she's prepared to engage with my service, please feel free to re-refer her. Yours, etc., Josie Singleton, Specialist Nurse, Diabetic Day Care Centre...'

Guess who. Becca Bagnet, that's who.

I did a quick check of her medical record. Sixteen in three months: until then, she's a minor. One quick tussle with the ethics of patient confidentiality later I was on the phone to her house. Her mother Claire picked up.

'Hello, it's Dr Copperfield from Bleak House... Fine thanks. Oh, good. Listen, I hate to play the heavy, but I've still got Becca's repeat prescription chart on my desk waiting to be updated and I *still* haven't got the results of the blood tests I asked for weeks ago. Do you happen to know whether she's had them done yet?'

What followed really came as no surprise.

Mum and dad were pretty much at the end of their tethers. Becca was coming home at all hours, if she came home at all. She was injecting herself with insulin pretty much at random, her clothes were hanging off her and you'd have thought, judging by the amount of time she spent in the bathroom with the radio blaring, that she'd look and smell better than she did.

If Claire could persuade her to come and see me, she would. Meanwhile, with her 'I've left my insulin prescription at home...' routine doing the business at GP practices all across town, I reckoned it would be quite a while before our paths crossed again.

THE TALENTED MR NICKLEBY

'I'VE STILL GOT that buzzing in my ear.'

Oh. My. God.

Here we go again.

'I'd like my cholesterol checked.'

I shouldn't rise to the bait of knight's move logic like this, but sometimes you can't help yourself.

'Why, when your problem's buzzing in your ear, do you want a cholesterol test?'

'Because I thought it might be the cause.'

I spent the next ten minutes unpicking this. I explained that high cholesterol causes no symptoms and that, therefore, it could not be the explanation for his symptoms, even if his cholesterol was elevated. That it is a risk factor – one of many – for heart disease and stroke, which were not items currently on our agenda, in that they were also not known to produce buzzing in the ears or any of his other multifarious symptoms. That treatment, if required, usually boils down to pills. That pills – according to his voluminous records and to his frequent protestations – never agree with him. And that, because of all the above, there was absolutely no reason to consider having a cholesterol test.

I spoke for around five minutes, and when I finished, I felt quite exhausted. There was a pause. I raised my eyebrows in a way which I hope conveyed that we were done.

He wasn't.

'So, are you going to check my cholesterol or not?' he said.

PORK PIE WEEK

'AH, TONY!' said our practice manager, Gruppenführer Jane Carstone. 'Just the man I wanted to see!'

I groaned, inwardly.

'Why are you groaning?' she said, sharply. 'I haven't told you what the problem is yet.'

Well, I *meant* it to be inward.

'Sorry,' I said. 'I… er…'

'Stop burbling and pull yourself together,' she said.

Jane isn't a partner in the business, or a doctor, but she is hideously switched on, and the sight of her bearing down on you with a clipboard is enough to make you burble. Inevitably, you're in trouble – you've filled in some forms incorrectly, parked in the Senior Partner's space, killed a patient, that sort of thing.

'Now,' she said, 'You're behind with your blood tests. There are a huge number of them in your inbox, and they need to be dealt with. I'll be raising it at the monthly partnership meeting next Monday.'

Every morning when I sit down at my desk there's an annoying icon flashing on my computer screen. It's the equivalent of the 'You've Got Mail!' message, but it means 'You've Got Test Results!' Yahoo! There are normally two or three dozen arriving each day and they need to be checked, commented on, actioned and then filed away in the patient's medical record.

Sounds easy enough? It would be, if all the results were from tests that I'd ordered on patients that I know – frankly, those are pretty easy to deal with. But a minority will be tests ordered by doctors who are away on holiday, on patients that I've never seen. Faced with the results of, say, some random liver checks, it's impossible to make a rational judgement without checking the patient's medical record and the results of any previous investigations.

Luckily, the NHS's fabulous IT systems make this a piece of cake. Ah, I nearly had you going there didn't I? Not only are the results buried under piles of computer-generated blanketry, but it's not possible to see the original request form setting out why the tests were asked for. Finding out that Mr Hexam's liver function tests are mildly abnormal as a side effect of the statin drug he's taking to lower his cholesterol, which is also slightly raised but better than it was when it was last measured, takes ages, and meanwhile the crowd outside in the waiting room is getting restless.

But needs must when the drivel drives.

'Well, you know I've been on holiday, Jane,' I said. 'There aren't that many of them but... look, I'll get on with it.'

'Good,' she said, turning to go. Then she paused. 'Oh, and Raynaud's and Scleroderma Awareness Week starts on Monday, too. I'm going to ask Mrs Peggotty to direct any fallout to you. Is that OK?'

The way the question was put, the only answer was Yes, so I said nothing. She stalked away, her heels click-clacking on the wooden floor.

Weird. I thought it was Ovarian Cancer Awareness? Or Mouth Cancer? Or Stroke Awareness? Maybe not. I wandered to my room, safe in the knowledge that one in three people I see over the next fortnight will be convinced they have Raynaud's Disease (a vascular disorder that affects blood flow to the fingers, toes, nose and ears when exposed to cold or in times of psychological stress).

Sure enough, there it was on the calendar above my desk – along with hundreds of other health campaigns of one sort or another, often overlapping.

The first week in May featured an ugly clash involving ME, psoriasis, epilepsy and allergy. I imagined being confronted by someone convinced they were suffering from the lot. At least it's also the start of National Smile Week.

The thing about all of this is that it is counter-productive: awareness isn't the same as understanding, and it's all part of why you have to wait ages for an appointment and can only have 10 minutes when you get one, and why I have to plough through endless surgeries of the worried well. My antipathy is shared by most doctors, who will tell you that a large number of their patients are only *too* aware of their own health, or perceived lack of it.

Mouth Cancer Week will transform simple ulcers into complex neuroses; Prostate Cancer Week will see floods of men worried about their trickling urinary stream; Migraine Week will leave me with a stonking headache; Gut Week – yes, really – will cater for those who can't even conjure up a proper symptom but who think, hell, I've got 22ft of gut, there must be *something* wrong there *somewhere*.

And for every early diagnosis there are hundreds of false alarms where we don't just raise awareness, but anxiety.

I tried pointing this out to the health centre staff last year when they wanted to force everyone to bedeck themselves with pink ribbons to mark Breast Awareness Month. It fell on deaf ears: this year they're all planning to dress from head to toe in pink. Next year? Presumably they paint the whole building. After that? God knows.

Of course, this absurd monster is mostly just a creation of PR companies and charities, with the willing compliance of NHS bureaucrats who don't understand medicine and think the millions splurged every year on poster campaigns is money well spent. Not long back, Sami Patel sent a letter to the PCT asking whether it was his imagination, or had Premature Ejaculation Day come early that year? My own preferred solution would be to retaliate with a campaign of our own – one promoting health obliviousness. We'd march through the streets chanting that we'd never heard of breast cancer, were unaware that most accidents occur in the home and that we believed it's normal to pass blood in our stools. Then we'd repair to the pub for some booze, a pork pie and a fag.

DIORALYTE

NICE – the National Institute for Clinical Excellence – isn't known for putting out helpful press releases, so it came as a pleasant surprise when it recently came up with some good advice for parents: don't run to your GP at the first sign of junior's squits. The symptoms can continue for up to two weeks with no sinister cause, they said, so don't worry your pretty little heads (or mine) about it until a fortnight has elapsed, so long as your diarrhoeal progeny are OK in themselves.

This was all ruined in the next breath when NICE added: 'And by the way, don't let your kids drink flat Coke as a remedy, because it doesn't work. You need to get some oral rehydration solution (ORS) down their necks, instead.'

Hang on, based on what evidence? I'm no anecdotalist, but I've been advising that particular homespun remedy for 20-odd years, and I can't remember the last time I admitted a dehydrated toddler. (The dehydration caused by constantly ejecting a stream of liquid from both ends of the body is the chief danger from gastroenteritis.)

The fact is, there is no evidence that flat Coke (or lemonade, or plain old squash) are no good. In fact, there are no studies looking at the effectiveness of fluids other than ORS in childhood gastroenteritis. So, the logic goes, stop using them, and use ORS instead. Bang goes many years' worth of clinical experience and observation.

The result? Parents clogging up the emergency surgery to get a tanker-load of Dioralyte or similar free on prescription – liquids, I might add, which are a hell of a lot harder to get down a whingeing toddler than two-day-old Coca Cola.

ANNOYING, PSEUDOSCIENTIFIC, QUASI-RELIGIOUS BAGGAGE

'DOCTOR,' SAID Mrs Garland, a slightly overweight lady wearing a tie-dye t-shirt, enormous hoop earrings and too many beads. 'I'm taking tincture of variegated Tasmanian clover leaf for my arthritis. I just wanted to check – is that OK?'

OK as in, will it make you better?

OK as in, will it destroy your liver?

Or OK as in, do I mind the implication that my conventional medical efforts at curing your dodgy knee are so ineffectual that you'll take your chances chewing on a random plant?

'Well,' I said. 'That… er… that depends.'

Complementary medicine is where the real money is.

The *smart* money goes on a decent stash of unbranded ibuprofen and some antiseptic to keep in the bathroom cabinet, but complementary medicine is where the big money is: the sort spent by one patient of mine who declared, without irony, that he had tried to cure his dog phobia with 'bark remedy'.

On my consulting room desk you'll find a bulky paperback entitled *Clinical Evidence*. This summarises the exhaustive research into everyday medical conditions.

I like to put the risks and benefits of treatments into some sort of context, and to do that I need evidence – data from clinical trials, involving patients and doctors who didn't know whether a live drug or an inert copy was being taken, and where the sample was large enough to demonstrate a difference in outcome, if one existed.

The evidence shows that conventional medicines are nowhere near as effective as I'd like them to be, true. But it also suggests that alternative therapies are often useless, overpriced cack.

That's not to say they all are. Some serious doctors cite scientific evidence supporting the use of butcher's broom, devil's claw and the Indian curry tree leaf for various conditions. (In the world of herbalism, a ridiculous name is no bar to therapeutic success.) St John's wort has long been used to treat mild depression, and saw palmetto prostate problems; they are so widely accepted by the medical fraternity that they occupy a distinct, if grey, area on the pharmacological map – a herbaceous border somewhere between conventional drugs and dodgy plant potions. And don't forget that about a quarter of prescription drugs, including hardy perennials such as aspirin and digoxin, are derived from plants.

The best thing about herbal medicine, though, is that it provides an ideal dumping ground for frequent attenders who make GPs want to resign whenever we see their names on our appointment lists – people who refuse to accept that there's nothing really wrong with them, for whom diverting them into the arms of a complementary therapist who won't actively harm them offers a solution.

Which rather raises the question: why does the mention of tincture of variegated Tasmanian clover leaf evoke in me (and most average GPs) a feeling normally reserved for when I've just trodden in something unsavoury?

First, because herbalism is generally taken far too seriously. We'll acknowledge that a few herbal treatments do the business if you'll admit that the rest are a load of nonsense.

Second, let's cut out all that annoying pseudoscientific, quasi-religious baggage, shall we? Apparently, many herbalists treat 'the whole person' by 'stimulating the body's natural healing powers' using cures derived, typically, from the 'mystic east'. Curing a snotty nose with a decongestant dispensed by a chemist in Herecaster clearly does not carry the same gravitas.

And third, let's recognise that, at times, herbalists do spout garbage at the gullible. For example, their cop-out treatment, when the random-herb-generator fails them, is always the same: listen to a herbalist for long enough and, inevitably, he will recommend camomile tea. This, it seems, cures everything from piles to psychosis.

Of course, the real issue with herbal treatments is that we GPs simply don't know enough about them to feel comfortable, or sound authoritative, with our herbivorous patients. Not through ignorance, or disinterest – it's just that the evidence required to give sensible advice isn't available.

While the *British National Formulary* bails me out of any standard prescribing conundrum, *Dr Hessayon's Vegetable and Herb Expert* still leaves me clueless on the beaded and be-hooped Mrs Garland's question of whether tincture of variegated Tasmanian clover leaf is OK.

Maybe it is, but I doubt it's as good as camomile tea.

CONCORDE

MRS Mann visited me yesterday, dragging her embarrassed husband with her. He sat in the chair opposite me, looking like a Bassett hound caught peeing on the carpet, while she talked on his behalf.

'It's his snoring,' she said. 'It's driving me round the bend. I haven't had a good night's sleep since... well, since I don't know when. He sounds like Concorde. You've got to do something about it before I brain him.'

'Like Concorde?' I said, sceptically.

'Like Concorde,' she said, whipping out a mobile phone as she spoke. 'I knew you wouldn't believe me, so I recorded him last night. I've set it as my ring tone.'

She pressed a couple of buttons, and the sound of Mr Mann's night-time rumblings issued forth. It did, indeed, sound like Concorde. My eyes widened in surprise.

'Told you,' she said, switching the phone back off and returning it to her handbag. She shot a withering glance at the man of her dreams. 'Now, what are you going to do about him?'

I looked at Mr Mann. He was approximately the size and shape of a walrus; therein probably lay a large part of the problem.

'Does he snore constantly at night?' I said.

'No,' said Mrs Mann. 'He snores for a few minutes, then he snorts and wakes up, and then he goes back to sleep and starts snoring again. Then he snorts and wakes up again. And that goes on and on. All night long.' She punctuated her speech by slapping her hand on my desk. 'I'm going to do him a bloody injustice one of these nights.'

'Hmmm,' I said. 'And is he tired during the day?'

'Is *he* tired during the day?' screeched Mrs Mann in indignation. 'I'm the one who's bloody tired!'

I decided to address Mr Mann directly. 'Would you say you're tired during the day?' I said.

'Tired?' he said. 'I'm too knackered to be tired.'

He eyed his wife nervously. She was looking at him with a venom bordering on the psychotic.

'Well,' I said, in my best, cheery let's-all-get-along voice. 'I think Mr Mann may be suffering from a thing called sleep apnoea. A lot of really serious snorers do. It's a condition in which the muscles and tissue of the throat relax as the patient falls asleep, closing off the airway momentarily. The brain gets starved of oxygen, and sends frantic messages which wake the person up. He splutters back to life and the whole cycle starts again. It can be quite deleterious...' Mrs Mann shot me a suspicious look. '...that is to say, quite *bad*, for the sufferer.'

In fact, people with sleep apnoea are so zonked out that they have an alarming tendency to fall asleep at the wheel, so in the long run evolution will wipe them all out. On the downside, they'll take quite a few of us with them.

'There are various types of sleep apnoea,' I said. 'Some are worse than others. In some cases, surgery is required, but I think you probably have a less severe form, Mr Mann. Do you drink?'

'A bit.'

'How much?'

'Say five or six cans a night. While I'm watching the telly and that.'

'Hmmm. I see. And do you smoke?'

'A bit.'

'How much?'

'About twenty a day.'

'Hmmm.'

'And you're 58 years old? Well, people of your age, particularly men, and particularly men who smoke and drink and are overweight, are the main sufferers of sleep apnoea. So here's what you need to do. You need to stop smoking if you can, or at least smoke less and not in the evenings. You need to drink less and, again, not in the evenings – that will also stop you getting up in the night to the loo.' He had developed a glazed look, so I turned to his wife. 'Does he do that, Mrs Mann?'

'Twice a night, every night.'

130

'OK, the other thing you need to do is lose a bit of weight, Mr Mann,' I said.

He was 5ft 8in tall and 16st 10lb. Although my dog could tell he was obese, I worked out his Body Mass Index. The fat walrus came in at a BMI of 37 – thoroughly obese. Not quite morbidly so, but not far off.

'Yes,' I said, shaking my head ruefully. 'It's as I thought – you do need to lose a few pounds. It shouldn't be too hard – walk to the shops, eat a little less, drink a little less. If you do that, and you cut out the smoking and drinking in the evenings, the apnoea should disappear. It'll be sweet dreams all round.'

'How long will that take?' said Mrs Mann, sharply.

'Well, it shouldn't take too long if he follows my advice.'

'So what happens to me in the meantime? I need some sleepers.'

Ah, sleepers. In some ways it would be nice to dole out the flurazepam or zolpidem, just to get the Mrs Manns of this world out of the surgery, so I can edge closer to my coffee break. But while sedating the punters into submission has its attractions, it's not really on.

'Well,' I said, 'the thing is, sleeping pills are addictive and they have quite a few dodgy side-effects. Do you drink?'

'A bit,' she said, slightly defensively.

'How much?'

'A few glasses of Lambrini, maybe.'

'A few glasses?' exploded Mr Mann, swivelling round in his chair. The worm was turning. '*A few glasses*? You don't want to listen to a word she says, doctor. She drinks a bottle a night. At *least*.'

'I do not!' she said.

'You do!' he said.

'I do *not*!' she said again.

I stepped in. 'OK, well, either way… And do you smoke?'

131

'A bit.'

'How much?'

'About twenty a day.'

'Hmmm. Yes. And are you a big fan of daytime TV?'

'I like *Cash In The Attic*. And *Bargain Hunters*. Sometimes *Jeremy Kyle*.'

'And in the evenings?'

'Well, I like to watch *Murder She Wrote*. It's always on UKTV Drama.'

'And *The Inspector Lynley Mysteries*,' said Mr Mann. 'Come on, let's have the truth. And *Bergerac*. And *A Touch Of Frost*. And *Brit Cops: Zero Tolerance*. And bloody *Magnum, PI*. She loves that Tom Selleck.'

I intervened before things turned nasty. (Or nastier.) 'So you'd admit that you sit around quite a lot watching the box? You see, that's perhaps part of the problem, particularly if it's late night telly, it gets your mind whirring. You know what, Mrs Mann, I think you'd benefit from taking a little more exercise, too. You could go for walks together.' She bristled. 'Well, it doesn't *have* to be together. But just turn the telly off, go for a walk, and when you get back home, drink a little less Lambrini and cut the smoking out. I think you'll soon find you sleep a lot better. Try and get to bed at the same time each night – routine really helps. And you could always buy some earplugs, too.'

HOME VISIT

AFTER THE HORROR of the Manns, I picked up my bag and headed out to the trusty Nissan on a home visit to a lady with stomach pain.

But, you say, surely GPs don't do home visits any more?

Not strictly true. Yes, we try to avoid them, but sometimes circumstances conspire against us: I might be on my way to the surgery when a call comes through requesting an urgent home visit for a 22-year-old male who is 'vomiting and dehydrating' and who lives a minute's drive away. I can almost guarantee that the sufferer will be a hung-over piss artist who half-reheated some week-old pizza last night. All he really needs is a routine 'take some clear fluids and see me in the morning' phone call, but I might as well give him 'Gastroenteritis for Dummies' face-to-face, rather than bump up my mobile bill.

Besides, until you've felt the soles of your shoes stick to a hallway floor, skirted around piles of pet droppings on the stairs and pulled a curtain rail off the bedroom wall to allow sunlight to enter for the first time in years, you've no business calling yourself a front-line medic. I recall one trip to a flat on the edge of civilisation, where – somewhere in the stygian gloom, under a duvet held together only by the crusty stains of bodily fluids, among the beer cans, ashtrays and black T-shirts – lurked a sickly Goth youth with a stiff neck and an aversion to light, the strength of which was unusual even for him. Alongside, watching with a quizzical eye, lay an iguana: this was my first case of reptile-poo-transmitted salmonella meningitis.

I put my collar up against the spitting rain, dashed across the surgery car park and got in to my car. I looked at my watch as I started the engine. Just gone 6.15pm. The patient lived on the right side of town for me, so it wasn't too painful; I could deal with her stomach pain and then head home for a well-deserved glass of something dry and white, and the latest Jack Reacher novel.

I trundled out onto the road and headed off to Market Way. Fifteen minutes later, I was outside the house – a 1930s semi with a caravan in the driveway and a ridiculous leylandii blocking out the sky. I knocked on the door. It was opened by a harassed-looking woman in her early 40s.

'Mrs Peecher?' I said. 'Dr Copperfield.'

'Oh,' she said, with less enthusiasm than she might have shown. 'Yes. Can you wait in your car for half an hour? Only, he's here at the moment and I haven't got room for both of you.'

'Who's here?' I said.

'You know,' she said, nodding in the direction of a van parked across the road. 'The telly man. That's why I called you out.'

I looked at the van. 'I'm sorry,' I said, 'but I don't understand. You called me out because the telly man's here?'

'Yes.'

'Eh?'

'He's come to install our Sky. They don't give you an exact time, you see.'

'But what has the TV man got to do with... wait a minute. Are you saying that you called me out – as opposed to coming in to the surgery to be seen – because you had the man from Sky TV coming round and you couldn't leave the house because he couldn't say when he'd be here?'

'Yes, that's right,' she said. 'He's nearly finished. Can you wait in the car?'

'Look,' I said, 'home visits are for patients who are genuinely ill and who can neither make their own way, nor be brought, to the surgery by someone else. I don't care if you're waiting for the man from Sky, the man from Atlantis or the man from Del Monte.'

I didn't wait in the car. In fact I didn't wait at all. No one keeps Reacher waiting.

STUPID DOCTORS

SADLY, PATIENTS AREN'T alone in their stupidity.

Over the years, I've been responsible for many cock-ups, many of them actually occurring on home visits.

Usually it's merely mildly embarrassing – I've lost count of the times I have been unable to retrace my route from a patient's bedroom to the front door, so that I've been found some time later by a relative, as I wander around the place like a retarded rat in a maze. On one occasion, I coaxed a rather mangy dog from out of the front garden back into a patient's house and up the stairs on to his sickbed. The idea was that the sight of his threadbare mutt would cheer the chap up. Unfortunately, it wasn't his dog.

Back in the days when we did a lot of out-of-hours visits, patients with emergencies like a slightly runny nose or a bit of a headache could call me at home and get me to drive out to them to hand them the paracetamol which was sitting on the bedside table two feet away. It was great fun. I remember arriving home one night at gone 7.30pm, after a particularly trying day of vomiting, incontinent kids and smelly old folks, with plans to do nothing but veg out on the sofa and watch the whole of series one of *The Office*.

I found Mrs Copperfield luxuriating in a tub of Radox and belting out her rendition of *Nessun Dorma* – a rendition, I must say, that Puccini would not have recognised.

'Two calls,' she trilled, a little too gleefully for my liking.

She always insisted on helpfully taking their details and promising on my behalf that I would ring them back immediately on my arrival.

I grabbed the notebook by the phone and looked at the first page. Hah! Toothache! Sorry, wrong profession. Try again when you pop your appendix.

I turned the page for the second message. 'Mr Brown,' it said. There was a number, and nothing else.

'*Mr Brown*?' I hissed, as the caterwauling continued from upstairs, oblivious. 'You could have got a bit more detail.'

I punched the handset and waited for it to ring, tapping my fingers on the table and thinking about my priorities: a shower, supper and David Brent.

'Hello?'

'Ah, is that Mr Brown?' I said.

'Yes, it is.'

'It's Dr Copperfield, here. I'll just take a few details. Your first name?'

'Eh?' he said.

'Your first name?' I said. 'Can I have it? Your first name? Come on, come on, I haven't got all night.'

'Why do you want to know my first name?' he replied, with more than a hint of suspicion.

'Well, isn't it rather obvious?' I said.

'Not really,' he said. 'I mean, is it important?'

No, I thought. *I'll just hand whatever pills you need to you out of a big bag. Who needs to keep records?*

'Well, of course it's important.'

Not least because I don't visit people called Wayne or Kyle.

'But why?'

'Look,' I thundered, 'you've called the doctor, right? Don't you think you might at least extend me the courtesy of giving me your name? You know? Hmmm? For my notes?'

There was a pause.

'I did call you,' he replied. 'But that was a month ago. And it was about your guttering. You had a problem with a leak.'

I looked down at the message book. I had turned over two pages.

'Wrong Mr Brown,' I said. 'Terribly sorry to have disturbed you. Good night.'

Then I slammed the phone down, broke into the bathroom and turned the cold tap on full.

But today I managed to top all of these humiliations.

I took a call from one of our local nursing homes for a lady who was 'off her legs'. Such calls elicit an unpleasant Pavlovian reflex, for the simple reason that they're almost always crap. The symptoms of the barely sentient are Chinese-whispered amongst only slightly-more-sentient staff, to be presented to the doctor by someone who learned their logic and clarity at the School for Railway Tannoy Announcers – and who knows to end every message with, 'Straight away please.'

Given the interruption to afternoon surgery, and the likely shambles ahead, I managed to work myself up to a nicely explosive pitch of irritation *en route*. So Dr Copperfield had a menacing look as he strode purposefully and pompously into the nursing home.

I barked at the nearest member of staff. 'Where's Mrs Skiffins? I've been called out urgently to assess her?'

My lips curled nicely into a sneer with the word 'urgently', and I spent the next few moments refining my 'I'm an important doctor in a hurry, and you're a bunch of tossers' expression.

The staff looked at each other in confusion. One was eventually brave enough to speak. 'I'm sorry Dr Copperfield, I don't know anything about this. And I don't actually know where Mrs Skiffins is.'

I snapped. Two decades'-worth of suppressed, nursing home-induced vitriol erupted. 'Bloody hell!' I roared. 'This really takes the sodding Rich Tea! You drag me out of surgery for an emergency and you don't even know where the sodding patient is! You should be ashamed of yourselves, sitting around on your fat backsides while the rest of us are trying to hold the NHS together. This is a load of... of...' I scrabbled frantically for an appropriately blistering, expletive-loaded and irrefutable phrase. 'It's a load of arse,' I said, finally.

Then something rather took the wind out of my sails. Matron arrived and started looking, first quizzically, and then amusedly, at her patient records.

Finally, she broke it to me. 'I'm sorry doctor,' she said, with an voice that oozed compassion. 'But I think you're in the wrong nursing home. This is The Evergreen. Perhaps Mrs Skiffins lives at Rosemount?'

She led me gently by the elbow back to the front door, in a manner she'd long used, I could tell, with the dribbly and incontinent.

Later, I reflected on this incident and asked Sami Patel what he thought this all meant. I was hoping he'd say I was stressed, overworked, perhaps heading for burnout.

'Tony,' he said, 'This simply means you're a pillock.'

MR ENDELL AND HIS CORNUCOPIA OF ILLNESSES

HAVING MADE IT this far, you'll be able to guess how this story develops. But I'm going to tell it anyway.

Mr Endell, an elderly patient with diabetes, heart failure, atrial fibrillation and renal impairment, sat and cried in my surgery today. Not for the first time.

It wasn't his cornucopia of illnesses; this, in itself, is actually not a particularly remarkable combination.

It wasn't the fact that diabetes is depressing for him (*and* me): these days, diabetic care is like playing the stock market, in that we invest heavily in the disease, my interest rate falls, and their GFRs[1] and ejection fractions[2] eventually crash.

It isn't a general preponderance to tears, either. Mr Endell is a stoical sort, and very uncomplaining. (His compliance with treatment is impeccable, despite the fact that his drugs are administered with a shovel.)

So what is it that regularly drives this long-suffering, multipathological and polypharmaceutical man to despair?

Correct: the big building down the road staffed by white-coated clever docs.

He is currently expected to attend five different outpatient clinics.

This means that, instead of spending what remains of his life enjoying himself as best he can, he is wasting most of it travelling to, sitting in, returning from or pondering over outpatient appointments. So many and varied are his hospital interactions and their various epiphenomena that he no longer has a social diary. He has an appointment book.

Every time he attends the hospital he winds up being seen by a different junior doctor, usually an earnest and enthusiastic trainee with one eye on him, one eye on that pretty blonde nurse and a third eye on the pub, who will never see him again and who randomly changes his medication. As a result of which, I've given up rewriting Mr Endell's repeat prescription card. Instead, I've just scrawled on it, 'Lots of drugs, PRN'. (From the Latin *pro re nata*, meaning 'when necessary'.)

Each hospital appointment generates another test which is carefully arranged so that the results won't be available for his follow-up visit. Or, if they have miraculously appeared, then his notes are missing, so the outcome is the same: a further follow-up appointment arranged by a hospital doctor who's annoyed at having had his time wasted and who doesn't mind letting my entirely innocent patient know.

Each clinic consultation is a mess of non-sequiturs, partial explanations, dysfunction, repetition, omission and miscommunication. I used to think that patients enduring secondary care suffered because the right hand didn't know what the left was doing. Now it's much worse. The hospital has turned into an octopus, and none of the eight arms have a clue what the other seven are up to. They only work in unison when they engulf the patient and drown him in 'care'.

I suspect people have been driven to murder for less. Frankly, if I were Mr Endell, I would hire a light aircraft and drop napalm on the consultants' car park. (Though, given that it's not entirely their fault, but that of the system they work in, maybe I'd strafe the managers' canteen, too.)

Instead, being a reasonable chap, he simply books an appointment with me to see if I can make any sense of it all.

But most times I haven't received the latest correspondence, and if I have, I can only marvel at the disintegration of care and how so many words can convey so little useful information.

I enjoy these consultations as much as I enjoy having needles stabbed in my eye; God *knows* what they're like for him.

Hospitals used to have 'general physicians'. These were specialists who weren't straitjacketed into a narrow field of interest like most modern consultants but who dabbled in lots of different areas – like, say, diabetes, heart failure, atrial fibrillation and renal impairment. They would have dealt with chaps like Mr Endell, and all the other patients who had baffled the hell out of me but who didn't fit into any neat category, such as people with intractable tiredness or non-specific dizziness. The great thing about them was that they tended to retain an overview of the 'whole person', unlike most typical modern-day 'narrow' specialists, who see the patient more as slices of discrete pathology, and deal only with their bit.

Unfortunately, the general physician has all but died out because of the trend to super-specialise and artificially compartmentalise medicine, and the ever-present default option of thinking the GP can deal with everything (usually we can, but occasionally we can't). The campaign to save our few remaining general physicians (and bring back more of them) starts here.

[1]GFRs (Glomerular Filtration Rates). Your kidneys are designed to filter your blood and remove the bad stuff; GFR is a measurement of how good a job they are doing.

[2]Ejection fractions: The percentage of blood pushed out of the heart's two pumping chambers, the left and right ventricles, when it contracts. A healthy heart pumps out more than half of the blood in the chamber. Excessively low ejection fractions indicate cardiac dodginess.

MORE ON MORON HOSPITALS

SADLY, MR ENDELL'S case is by no means unusual.

Hospitals are dodgy places at the best of times. In-patients suffer triple jeopardy from antibiotic-resistant germs, bowel-obsessed nurses and doctors who do inappropriate tests to justify unnecessary treatments. Also, the food's terrible. But these all pale into insignificance compared with the appointment dysfunction which secondary care applies to screw up our patients' lives.

Forget waiting lists – they're just a minor irritant by comparison. Appointment dysfunction really messes with the punters' minds: their hopes are raised then dashed, their arrangements callously disregarded and their attempts at resolution thwarted at every turn. Book an outpatient appointment and you're sending them on a one-way journey to hell.

If you think I'm exaggerating, ask your own GPs. If they're honest, they'll say that a quarter of their current workload stems from hospital-based appointment cock-ups. Here are some examples from my own recent practice:

- A young man has his CT scan, but his follow-up slot is postponed three times. Unsurprisingly, his headaches are getting worse.
- A woman receives a snotty note from her specialist discharging her because she didn't attend an ultrasound scan. Which was hardly surprising, as the appointment was sent to the wrong address.
- An elderly man is told he needs an echocardiogram with a subsequent cardiology follow-up appointment. Predictably, the date for the latter precedes the former – and his attempts to postpone the echo result in him being taken off the list for both.
- A man with carcinoma of the prostate has his three-monthly Zoladex implant appointment postponed indefinitely, with no advice about rearranging his ongoing treatment.

I could go on, but I don't need to. GPs encounter these absurdities every day. Strictly speaking, we *could* tell the punters to bog off – we've done our bit, and the issue lies between them and the hospital. But these patients are terminally exasperated and I'm on their side. Once in the system, they enter a Kafka-esque nightmare where they can get no help, no answers and no sense. And all the while, in many cases, the fear and uncertainty puts normal life on hold.

I'm probably feeling sympathetic because I had a dose of dysfunction myself recently, when I tried to arrange an urgent appointment for a Mr Heep. He was suffering cardiac-sounding chest pain – not quite bad enough to send him in as an emergency, but bad enough that firing off a standard referral would have left me uneasy, and quite possibly waking in the night in a cold sweat.

I spoke to the duty medical registrar at the hospital.

'If I were you I would refer him to the Rapid Access Chest Pain Clinic,' she said.

Fine. Except, a few days later, I received a call from that clinic. 'It's about your Mr Heep,' said the caller. 'Only he doesn't seem to fit our criteria. He's actually too urgent for us and I think you should send him in to hospital.'

Once locked into these circular nightmares, there is a grave danger of the GP needing a referral, too – to a proctologist, because, after going round in so many circles, I'll have disappeared up my own bottom.

Of course, dealing with the hospital appointment system has always involved banging your head against a brick wall. But this episode illustrates that the protocol mentality, automated systems and slick technology of the brave new NHS have served only to make that wall harder and higher. And it's damaging the brains of those who have to use it.

Until someone sorts it out, the only thing I can suggest is to lower patients' expectations of the system. How? Simply rebadge the outpatient slot with the prefix, 'dis'. As in, 'I'm sorry, I'm going to have to book you a disappointment at the hospital.' Because that's what they're going to get.

YET MORE MR NICKLEBY

'I'VE STILL GOT that buzzing in my ear.'

'And?'

'And I saw your young Dr Lucie the other day and she checked my blood pressure. She said it was up, she did, and said I needed to come and see you.'

I made a mental note to box young Dr Lucie's ears next time I saw her. Never, *EVER*, check a heartsink's blood pressure. That way madness lies. It's bound to be up, and the news will only exacerbate the spiral of anxiety and so perpetuate our mutual agony. Besides, the idea of checking blood pressure is, ultimately, to save lives. And, where heartsinks are concerned, that rather seems to go against natural evolutionary processes.

So… we reprised the cholesterol conversation of some time ago, with the same negligible level of success. Wearily, I checked his blood pressure myself and declared it to be normal.

I thought to myself, *If he says, 'So what's causing this buzzing in my ear, then?' I shall scream.*

'So what's causing this buzzing in my ear, then?' he said.

THE NUMBER NEEDED TO TREAT

UNLIKE MR NICKLEBY, many patients have a massive and almost entirely unjustifiable faith in modern medicines.

Maybe that isn't surprising when you consider that some of them also think that having their feet massaged will detox their liver and that crystal healing will settle the symptoms of their arthritis. Given a cast iron diagnosis such as a proven urinary infection (where you've actually grown the infecting bacteria on a Petri dish), most people would assume that every patient treated would get better sooner after a course of antibiotics. In fact, even if the antibiotic appears to kill off the germ in the lab, only one patient in every four that takes the tablets gets better any more quickly than if they'd just taken lots of clear fluids.

Put another way, four people have to be treated to obtain benefit for one, a statistical concept known as the Number Needed to Treat, or NNT.

Doctors have been calculating and using NNTs for about 20 years now, and the results are nowhere near as favourable as patients might expect. To quote a fairly well-known example, 85 patients have to take a cholesterol-lowering drug for five years to prevent one heart attack. Now that the most popular cholesterol-lowering drug, simvastatin, is out of patent and costs the NHS around £1 per patient per month, treating the other 84 is obviously cost effective. But when statins cost £1 per patient per day – as they did when they first appeared – the health economists could argue the case against prescribing them in all but the most severe cases.

And these numbers take no account of any side effects that the patients might suffer along the way. Department store magnate John Wanamaker famously complained that half the money he spent on advertising was wasted. He had it easy. If I invented a drug that helped half the people who took it, and harmed none of the others, I'd be in Nobel prize territory.

THE MARKET FOR KNOCKED-OFF OPHTHALMOSCOPES

IT SNOWED THIS MORNING, which at least covered up the chewing gum and dog mess plastered on the pavement outside the practice entrance. Tomorrow it will be brownish-grey sludge, but today it looked quite nice.

I parked in front of one of the big steel security doors locking off the area where they deliver all our drugs and liquid nitrogen. It probably wouldn't be sensible to walk through the main doors carrying big boxes labelled 'Opiate-Based Analgaesics', but I've often thought we could employ the liquid nitrogen (for freezing off warts) in reception. A bit of dry ice floating about would make for a nice dramatic start to the day – maybe with some strobes thrown in to liven up the epileptics.

The two steel doors were covered in graffiti tags and I noticed a new line had been added: 'KYLE CHUZZLEWIT = STILL THE MAN'. Next to it, someone else had daubed the phrase '*Ping pong willy*'. I have no idea what that means. Is it a nickname, an STI or a novel way of playing table tennis?

In the waiting room, amid the usual mayhem, Mrs Peggotty grabbed me.

'Look at this, doctor,' she said.

She shoved a small cardboard box under my nose. I peered inside. A small rodent looked up at me.

'A small boy just threw it in and ran off,' said Mrs Peggotty.

It's a very odd thing, but our practice has long been a repository for unwanted local pets. We had a dog abandoned in the waiting room once. And a lady slipped a Siamese fighting fish into our aquarium. It gradually ate all the other fish, until it died; after that, we got rid of the aquarium.

'What is it?' I said.

'I think it's a hamster, but Tracey swears it's a gerbil and Gordon thinks it's a rat,' she said. 'I was thinking of taking it down to the vet. But do you think they'd… kill it?'

'I'm sure they'll treat it with the care with which we treat *our* patients, Mrs Peggotty,' I said.

I struggled past the teeming hordes of slightly poorly, worried well and downright hypochondriacs, dumped my briefcase in my room and then popped down to the gents for a pee.

In the corridor, I met the Senior Partner.

'Have you seen my ophthalmoscope?' he said, irritatedly. This is the instrument a doctor uses to examine your eye for things like glaucoma, retinal disease and brain tumours, while you each try not to gag on the other's bad breath.

'No, sorry,' I said. 'Lost another one, then?'

'Lost?' he snapped, stomping off. 'It's been bloody stolen.'

I wondered idly at the market for knocked-off ophthalmoscopes: it can't be huge. But then we're always getting stuff go walkabout from the practice. Stethoscopes regularly disappear – usually nicked by trainee doctors. Once we had an ear-syringing machine go. Why? What are they going to *do* with it? We used to get a lot of people wandering in from time to time and trying the doors to our consulting rooms. My camera was taken from a locked drawer, and lots of sets of car keys have been pinched over the years. One partner had his car stolen, too. Most embarrassingly, a year or two back we were all sitting in the common room eating lunch when a guy walked in, picked up the TV and walked out. We all assumed he was a repairman. Sami Patel even held the door open for him. Since that episode and the car, we decided to beef things up a bit more. Now all of our doors have electronic locks which open with a dongle (an electronic key). But we still have nice, big, ground floor windows which offer easy access to the more committed local scrotes.

I headed to the loo. Inside, the hot tap was trickling merrily away, as it has done for the last six months. We've mentioned it to the Trust a few times, but the same people who come down on you like a ton of bricks for using a Drug X instead of Drug Y which is threepence a dose cheaper don't seem to be concerned about us warming the drains of Clareshire. At the last partnership meeting, I offered to go to B&Q, buy a new tap and some washers, come in with my tools and fix the bloody thing myself. But Obergruppenführer Jane Carstone would have none of it: think of the health and safety issues!

It's not as though I'm not competent. I once fixed a patient's toilet. She was an old lady who called me out to her house for some minor ailment. While I was there, I noticed that her loo was running permanently. I immediately diagnosed a sinking ballcock, nipped out to my car for my adjustable spanner, took off the top of the cistern and fixed it.

'Oh, thanks doctor,' she said. 'I was going to call a plumber out, but there's no need now.'

It was the least I could do for her. In fact, it was *all* I could do for her.

COMPLAINTS

ON MONDAY THIS WEEK, a lady complimented me on my doctoring, at which point I fell off my chair in a dead faint and had to be revived by the Senior Partner.

Alright, when I say 'I fell off my chair', actually I just blinked in surprise. And when I say 'complimented', what she actually said was that she had resorted to seeing me because, and I quote, 'I've heard that you're marginally less crap than the rest of them.'

Still, I regarded this as quite a recommendation and immediately ordered a set of personalised stationery:

> *Dr Tony Copperfield MBBS MRCGP*
> *'Marginally Less Crap Than The Rest Of Them'*

I also inserted a note of this 'patient feedback' into my files, ready for the annual 'appraisal' which I was about to undergo.

Later that day I saw Mr Walker. The chances of getting a 'thank you' out of him are about on a par with the Department of Health doing something sensible to help doctors (or patients), so his name on my computer screen did not fill my heart with joy. He is perhaps our Numero Uno complainer – and God knows we've got a few of them. Almost every consultation seems to begin or end, or sometimes both, with a whinge about something. Among the more recent have been that the magazines in the waiting room are boring, that there aren't enough car parking spaces and that I looked up a drug dose in the textbook before issuing a prescription (perhaps he'd prefer that I hazard a guess? I know I would.).

The funny thing about Mr Walker is that there are usually plenty of things about *him* which are worthy of complaint, too – from his body odour to his sheer irrelevance; if only we had a procedure for complaining about patients – that would make life more interesting.

This time, he turned up 10 minutes late for a 10 minute appointment.

You don't need to be Einstein etc etc. Still, that didn't stop him barging in and demanding to be seen.

'I think you're taking the mickey a bit here, Mr Walker,' I said. 'I'm afraid I can't see you now because that would mean that other people who have taken the trouble to arrive on time would have to wait. If you go back to the waiting room, I'll see you during my lunch break at midday.'

He was grievously offended by this. I know that because when he got home later he was kind enough to take time out of his busy schedule to write to Polizeiführer Jane Carstone about it in a letter which arrived this morning. If he had an excuse for being late, he didn't mention it, either at the time or in his letter. Ironically, by the time he came back in to see me at noon, he spent the first five minutes moaning about how difficult it had been to get the appointment in the first place. He would have used up the rest of his time bad-mouthing the NHS in general and GPs in particular if I hadn't skilfully directed the conversation on to the subject of his pressing need for medical care by using one of those tried and tested stock phrases from *The Real Life GP's Workbook*: 'Get to the bloody point then, my lunch is waiting.'

Complaints are big business in the NHS, actually. Not long ago, the Healthcare Commission published a study into how well the organisation deals with criticism, and decided that there was room for improvement. It said that patients wanted their grievances to be dealt with quickly – which, as any NHS employee knows, translates to: 'We'd like our compensation cheques by return of post.'

It also claimed that relatives primarily wanted 'reassurance' that changes would be made only in order that 'other innocent families wouldn't suffer in the way that they had'.

In English: 'We'd rather have it in cash if poss?'

The Patients' Association thinks that doctors don't welcome feedback from patients. They couldn't be more wrong; we love it. Taking pride of place on the 'dumb complaint of the week' notice board in our common room is a letter breaking the news that 'Dr Copperfield squeezes his patients' testicles'. It's true – I've even been known to give my own a tweak during a particularly tedious consultation, just to stay awake – but then I also squeeze people's boobs, buttocks, armpits, groins, *labia majorae*, ear lobes, necks and those funny hollows behind their knees. Anywhere, in fact, where a suspicious lump might be found.

The Healthcare Commission further suggested that NHS Trusts should make it easier for patients to complain, by allowing verbal as well as written submissions. Yesterday one cheeky little tyke called our practice nurse Susie a 'clumsy bitch' after his pre-school immunisation; perhaps we should have treated this as a formal verbal complaint? After all, if we wait until he learns to read and write, his complaint will be judged to be out-of-time and dismissed without further investigation. And we can't have that.

The biggest grievance from patients generally is that GPs rush them. They might have a point. Since I was a fluffy trainee, the time allocated for routine appointments has increased from seven minutes to ten. However, the extra time has been more than swallowed up by the ever-growing and compulsory paperwork that forms part of most consultations. By the time I've ticked all those government-mandated QOF boxes by nagging you about smoking, drinking, eating too much, eating too little, using a sunbed, not using a condom, and have taken your blood pressure, measured your height, weight and waistline, checked your urine for sugar and asked whether you felt like topping yourself recently, it's almost time to push the button that lights up the 'Next patient please' sign outside the door.

Whatever you actually wanted to see me about will have to squeeze into the remaining 90 seconds, or wait until next time – unless, of course, you actually are an obese, malnourished, nicotine-addicted diabetic melancholic alcoholic with an all-over tan and a burning sensation when you pee, in which case you've absolutely come to the right place.

All that said, considering that we spend most of our time sticking sharp things into people and telling them to stop doing things they enjoy, we get surprisingly few moans. Every year there are almost

400 million patient contacts, and last year they gave rise to 140,000 complaints. Ten thousand of those were referred to the Commission and, of those, one in five was considered justifiable. So: 2,000 justifiable complaints out of 400 million appointments. By my maths, that's 200,000:1. For the average GP working 48 hours a week, that equates to about 15 years' worth of face-to-face consultations for every dropped (or squeezed) bollock.

At going home time, I nipped into the common room and pinned Mr Walker's letter up on the notice board next to all the over-underlined, green inked notes. The head receptionist Mrs Peggotty was in there, and she collared me.

'Oh, there you are, Dr Copperfield,' she said, bustling over, a touching look of motherly concern on her face. 'Now then, you know Mrs Wemmick who you saw yesterday?'

'Mrs Wemmick?' I said. 'Ah, yes. Thirties, slightly anaemic. Asked me for my name after the appointment, even though it's written on my door in big capital letters. A complaint, I suppose?'

'Oh, quite the reverse, doctor,' said Mrs Peggotty, brandishing a spangled plastic bag. 'She brought this in for you. Only, what on earth shall I *do* about it?'

I peered inside the bag. Blimey! Another thank you! This time a written one, on a card! With a bottle of Chilean merlot!

I'm not surprised Mrs Peggotty didn't know what to do about it.

The NHS has a hierarchy in place to deal with complaints, but anything complimentary leaves everybody scratching their heads.

At the Royal Cornwall Hospital NHS trust, they introduced a 'chocolate audit', under which all presents given to staff must be logged as a proxy measure of patient satisfaction. Given that nurses already waste vast amounts of effort on paperwork – every time a patient opens his bowels it requires a case conference and the completion of an incident form – the only logical response is for ward staff to 'Just say no' to boxes of chocs from the grateful un-dead. They may feel unappreciated, but they'll have one less piece of bureaucracy to deal with.

In my case, it turned out that I am now obliged to write to Mrs Wemmick within seven working days, thanking her for taking the time to bring the matter of my good performance to my attention. I must assure her that the circumstances leading up to her flattering remarks will be fully investigated and that I will contact her again within two weeks outlining what steps the practice will take to prevent any recurrence.

Only when the issues have been fully investigated and the correspondence copied to the Primary Care Trust can I close the file. Or in this case, recycle the bottle. Cheers!

GOOD THINGS COME IN THREES

NO SOONER HAD I recovered from the shock of Mrs Wemmick's Chilean merlot (and the hangover) than *another* patient was at it.

Mrs Cobham was the daughter of an elderly lady whom I had treated over the years for a variety of ailments which had culminated in her death. That is to say, the ailments, and not my treatments, had led to this culmination.

The daughter booked an appointment, ostensibly to discuss her own varicose veins. But she soon cut to the chase.

'Look, doctor,' she said, bending down to rummage in a plastic bag at her feet. 'I just wanted to thank you for the way you looked after my mother.'

Being thanked is always an awkward and quite touching moment on the rare occasions it happens in person. And along with the warm glow of knowing that hey, at times, the doctor-patient relationship really *is* special, there is that pleasurable *frisson* of anticipation: maybe this time they've gone for The Big One!

I edged forward in my seat, craning my neck slightly but trying not to make it obvious.

Sadly, this was more solid than a cheque. Perhaps another bottle… only this time containing something fizzy and vintage, and conveniently just under the £100 threshhold*?

Mrs Cobham sat back up and plonked a plastic bag on the desk in front of me.

I was already preparing my protests: *Oh, you really shouldn't, it was the least I… well, if you insist…*

Excitedly, I peered into the bag. And from it, I removed something quite extraordinary: one loaf of sliced bread (white).

'We… I mean, the whole family, really… we wanted to show our appreciation for everything you did for mum,' she said, by way of explanation.

I was momentarily stuck dumb. I had treated her mother for the past 14 years, averaging one consultation a month. Ten minutes x 12 = 120 minutes, makes two hours a year, two hours x 14 makes… 28 hours. For which I receive, as a heartfelt thank you, one loaf of Warburton's 'Toastie', 400g. Not even the 800g daddy, note. Sell-by date, yesterday.

'Erm… thank you,' I heard myself say. 'That's… well, that's lovely.'

She nodded and smiled, sweetly. 'It was the least we could do,' she said.

You're not wrong there.

Later, my colleagues offered their own explanations for this incident.

Dr Emma clucked and cooed, and said 'Ah, bless!' a lot. 'I think they're trying to say that they think you're the best thing since… you know,' she said. 'Ah, how sweet! Isn't that lovely?'

Sami Patel scratched his head for a while and then said, 'Maybe someone told her to take some bread to the duck, and she misheard "ducks" for "docs"?' he said. 'That's the best I can do.'

The Senior Partner looked at me over his half moon specs. 'No,' he said. 'She has concluded, quite correctly, that that is all Copperfield is worth. In fact, I think she has erred on the side of generosity.'

The truth is that it was probably a last-minute decision *en route* to the appointment and all she had to hand. In which case it could just as easily have been a loofah, so perhaps I should count my blessings.

I believe present-giving has declined in the years I've been in practice. You might say that this is because I am a terrible disappointment to my patients, but my colleagues confirm the trend, and the consensus is that, these days, patients are just too busy writing letters of complaint about us to get to the shops.

Of course, there are those who try to bribe you with gifts. Last Christmas, a bloke who wanted a sick note for his highly tenuous back pain tried it on with a turkey (he got only a week, because it was small and unplucked), and some years ago I read a *Doctor* magazine survey in which one GP recounted how a patient placed a large white cabbage on to his desk, looked him in the eye and said, 'Do you think I need a scan, doc?' To which the only answer, surely, was 'If you think you can bribe me with a vegetable, yes.' But it's usually more subtle, like the pleasant but neurotic chap who calculated that the chances of my reading his 100-page internet print-out of all the alternative treatments for his stress-induced hives might be enhanced by the offer of a box of holiday fudge. (That didn't work either.) In the same *Doctor* mag survey, GPs submitted the worst presents they'd received from patients. Contenders included cans of deodorant, a bag of Brussels sprouts and a giant china Winnie-the-Pooh. The winners: a tie between a penis enlarger and a three-hour video of a patient playing the organ.

Of course, we GPs are highly unlikely to complain about such largesse. The job has few other perks, and our nurses and receptionists are delighted when we share our spoils. So, obviously, that's what I did with the bread.

* We have strict rules about what we can 'reasonably receive'. Specifically, we have to declare any gifts from patients or relatives worth more than £100, and those from pharmaceutical representatives valued above £6. I find it insulting to be the subject of such draconian scrutiny. The implication is that I might prescribe a certain product if the drug rep gives me a nice pen to sign the prescription with, or that I might be happy to bump off granny for the cost of filling my car with petrol. I won't and I'm not. On the other hand, if you're offering a week in Barbados…

APPRAISALS AND REVALIDATION

SAMI LOOKED CONFUSED as he walked into the common room. He watched me pour a coffee, and then said, 'Hang on… you're not here.'

'Clearly I am,' I said.

'Well, the appointment system says you're not. But if you are, shouldn't we book you some patients? I'll give reception a ring and…'

I held up my hand and pointed to a large pink folder sitting on the table in front of me.

The penny dropped. 'Ah, appraisal-cramming day,' he said. 'Well, at least you could look more cheerful about it.'

Maybe I could. But while there are many things I'd rather do than see another surgery load of the catarrhal and diarrhoeal – like, on a bad day, chew glass – preparing for my appraisal isn't one of them.

We GPs have had to suffer an annual appraisal since 2002, though it feels a lot longer. Beardy, sandal-wearing educationalists enthuse over the process and spout platitudes about it being 'facilitated self-reflection and challenged self-assessment'. The rest of us view it as a pain in the backside.

What, exactly, is appraisal? And how does it differ from revalidation, the other modern educationopolitical hot potato?

Every year, we GPs compile an 'Appraisal Folder' of information: practice activity data, audits, certificates of attendance at educational meetings, complaints and even the occasional thank you card from patients like Mrs Wemmick to show what we've been up to. Gathering all this stuff together, jumping through the inevitable hoops and ticking the bureaucratic boxes is mind-numbingly tedious and very time-consuming – hence the 'day off' to get it all done.

Worse than that, it's patronising and insulting.

Here's an example. Under the 'Maintaining good medical practice' section, we're supposed to collect PUNs and DENs. These are 'Patient's unmet needs' and 'Doctor's educational needs', for the uninitiated. Let me explain.

Dr C: 'Good morning, what can I do for you?'

Patient: 'Well, it's about these tattoos.' (He shows me the standard-issue Love/Hate on his knuckles).

Dr C: 'I see. What about them?'

Patient: 'I'm thinking of applying for a job in social services, so I'd like them removed. What's the best way of going about it?'

Dr C: 'Well, that's a good question. No-one has asked me for ages. Let's think. The last time I was involved in tattoo removal was… blimey… 26 years ago, when I was a surgical houseman. Yes… I was assisting at an emergency appendicectomy, and when the patient was under anaesthetic we noticed he had "Chelsea FC" tattooed on his penis.'

Patient: 'I see.'

Dr C: 'So we thought it would be a bit of a laugh if we tried to remove it. His tattoo, that is, not his penis. We got the scrub nurse to scrub it with all sorts. Nothing worked. Of course, this was in the days before we worried about things like consent.'

Patient: 'Right, so…'

Dr C: 'So you want to know how to get rid of your tattoo. And I'm not entirely sure of the best way to do it.' (Patient's unmet need.)

Patient: 'OK…'

Dr C: 'So I need to brush up my knowledge.' (Doctor's educational need. Brilliant, isn't it?) 'Which I'll do. Then I'll give you a ring.'

He won't get his tattoo removal on the NHS, but that's not the point. The point is that I'm supposed to 'log' every time I'm in PUN/DEN territory, so I can prove to my appraiser at our annual get-together that I think/learn/help out patients. This is crap, because general practice is so full of variety and surprise that *every* surgery prompts me to check this fact, that drug regime or the other NICE guidance. Not because I'm thick or amnesic, but because I want to do a good, up-to-date job. Plugging knowledge gaps to improve practice is what any self-respecting, motivated professional does *automatically*. I hate the assumption that without the appraisal's PUN and DEN prompt I might forget all about it. I hate the time spent creating a sodding PUN/DEN album. And I hate the fact that it's all dressed up in educational, acronymal jargon.

PUNs and DENs are just one teensy part of appraisal, of course, but you get the drift. So did my appraiser, because I scrawled 'conscientious objector' over much of the paperwork. And, after the statutory three-hour appraisal meeting, he wearily shook his head in resignation as he signed me up for another year.

Unbelievably, though, it's about to get worse.

Appraisal is supposed to be 'formative'. In other words, it helps us GPs 'develop' – though, in my case, the only thing it really develops are frown lines and a sense of despair.

But revalidation: that's 'summative'. It's appraisal with knobs on, or with teeth. It's the five-yearly process by which I will have to prove to the GMC that I'm still fit to practise. (Revalidation is supposed to kick in next year, but it has been due to start 'next year' for about as long as I can remember.)

The popular view is that it will help to prevent another Dr Shipman, though that's not the official GMC line – not least because Shipman might well have sailed through, on account of a dearth of questions such as, 'Have you murdered many of your patients lately, go on, tell us, honestly, have you?'

This is how it's supposed to work. To get my 'fit for purpose' rubber stamp, I will need my five years' worth of appraisals in a nice, gift-wrapped presentation pack; some patient surveys; multi-source feedback from colleagues; significant event audits; 200 learning credits (don't even ask); and, the way things are going, a week-long run on a West End stage of a self-penned rock opera depicting the working life of a GP ('We Will Doc You').

The amount of time and money this will suck out of the NHS is mind boggling, which is probably why it keeps getting postponed. The benefits, on the other hand, will be tiny.

I can understand the public finding it reassuring that GPs should get 'certified' every five years – it would be nice to know that, say, the man with his finger currently up your jacksie is Someone Who Knows What He's Doing.

But training to become a GP takes ten long, hard years. That in itself tells you something about those who come out the other end clutching their MRCGP (Membership of the Royal College of General Practitioners). Despite my cathartic moaning, it's a great job, and not one that we're going to want to screw up in a hurry – even if that means having to keep up to date by reading the odd journal and listening to the occasional lecture.

Besides, GPs are already scrutinised to within an inch of their lives. Concerned patients can complain to the PCT, the GMC or the nearest ambulance-chasing lawyer. The government has various and ever-changing quangos ready to do their 'ton of bricks' thing. Our QOF scores give an idea of how we're performing and are scrutinised via an annual visit. The PCTs themselves routinely collect all sorts of data on what we're up to. And so on and so forth.

The fact is, the suits and the clipboard brigade can already smell the bad apples. Why make the rest of us suffer by holding the double barrelled shotgun of appraisal and revalidation to our heads?

One thing's for sure. The key revalidation section, 'Describe your work', will be easy to complete: 'Preparing for this crap.' Remember that next time you can't get an appointment with your GP!

ABOUT THOSE DOCTORS AND THEIR EDUCATIONAL NEEDS

HERE'S A HEADLINE you'll never see: 'No more training required for GPs.'

After all, turn on the radio, switch on the TV or open the newspaper and, chances are, you'll see or hear, 'GPs need more training in depression/ADHD/phenylketonuria/[insert disease of the day here depending on which charity, health evangelist or awareness campaign has been banging its particular drum]'.

We hear this 'GPs need more training in…' mantra so often, and it's completely wrong.

Imagine you just limped into my surgery because, last night – during your GP-prescribed two mile blubber-busting jog – you turned over your ankle. Cue pain and swelling: a sprain.

I prod around to rule out a fracture, then I advise the time-honoured quartet of rest, ice, compression and elevation – maybe with some bonus anti-inflammatories thrown in. You'll get better in a couple of weeks.

Now imagine something different. Pretend that, somehow, you hobbled directly all the way to an orthopaedic consultant, without passing 'GP' – maybe you're his secretary's other half, so you snuck in under the radar. He'll prod around, like me, to exclude a fracture. Because it's his field, he'll rule out some fancy and obscure dislocation or other, too, which you won't have because it's so rare. He'll advise the RICE ritual, as I did – but he'll also pack you off for an X-ray or even a scan, to be on the safe side, plus some physiotherapy and maybe a rehab follow-up with a sports injury specialist.

The upshot? You get better in two weeks – minus, maybe, a day.

So here's the thing. You've not had such detailed or intensive care from me: I'm a generalist, not a specialist, remember, so let's say I'm working to the 90% level of perfection. The clever, white coated guy with the superior expression and the personalised parking space will give you the full-on 100% – but all that extra time, hassle and cost has only made one day's worth of difference.

This principle applies to countless other medical problems. You get the vast majority of benefit from your humble GP working to that 'good enough' level, while that last 10% is subject to the law of diminishing returns – a huge amount of effort for minimal benefit.

Of course, a few people really do need us to pitch for perfection, when they might be suffering something serious or incapacitating. That's the GP's cue to open the gate and let you have a thorough going-over at the local hospital.

Single issue health campaigners don't understand, or accept, this logic because they're blinkered by their own particular interest. Hence those headlines. GPs can't know everything about everything. But we can – and do – know something about everything. This means that, given the constraints of time and resources the NHS imposes on us, we Jacks of all Trades give you a deal that may be less than perfect, but is perfectly adequate. More training, though? No. Because the better I become in any one area, the worse a generalist I am.

REBECCA BAGNET
PUSHES IT TOO FAR

IN OUR SUMPTUOUSLY-FURNISHED coffee room you'll find the Big Board. Named after the display screens in the War Room in Kubrick's brilliant *Dr Strangelove*, the Big Board is where you'll find the 'Dumbassed Complaint of the Month' letter, the practice's weekly timetable, names of patients who are currently receiving terminal care services at home, a list of recent deaths (both patient and celebrity, the latter copied from Wikipedia) and a list of current hospital in-patients, as advised by our local A&E departments.

This morning I noticed that Rebecca Bagnet's name had been added to the in-patient list.

She was currently residing in the Intensive Care Unit at Clareshire University Hospital. A phone call to the hospital switchboard got me precisely nowhere. Luckily, one of our recent trainees was currently wandering the wards as a junior doctor. I got the switchboard to fast bleep her.

'Stephanie? Hi, it's Tony. Tony Copperfield from Bleak House. I just wondered...'

Becca had been admitted two nights earlier, on her 16th birthday. She'd missed an insulin dose or two, necked a few celebratory Breezers, and was halfway through a piece of cake when she hit the deck. Her mates, who were getting used to this by now, tried the glucose syrup trick, but when the paramedics arrived they found her blood sugar wasn't too *low*, as it usually was, but far too *high*.

A combination of missed insulin, alcohol, icing sugar and an infection around a recent piercing (lower lip, as it happened) had tipped her into DKA, diabetic keto-acidotic coma, with a side order of septicaemia.

Mum and Dad were pulling shifts at the cot side.

'I'm assuming her biochemistry was up the spout, Steph?'

'Hey, and they say GPs know nothing about physiology...'

'Stop playing the white coated cynic and listen up for a second. I think there's another reason why her acid/alkali balance is way off – I'm pretty sure she's bingeing and vomiting and losing stomach acid as a result. You could check the enamel on her teeth for signs of acid damage.'

'She's being ventilated, Tony. I don't think I'd get much of a view.'

'Just the same, when she comes round, could you ask the liaison psychiatrist to do the warm, non-threatening, fluffy bunny routine?'

'It's an "if", Tony, not a "when". She's on the "Five Tube" list. A visit from the Freud Squad isn't exactly a high priority at the moment.'

This is serious stuff. Where patients have tubes going into or out of five or more orifices, this is prognostically equivalent to the Grim Reaper enquiring about visiting hours. The ITU guys weren't giving up hope just yet, but they were checking her handbag for donor cards and they weren't buying her any DVD box sets. But hey – spending your 16th birthday in intensive care... how cool is that?

A WALKING STICK TO BEAT YOU WITH

I'M A MILD-MANNERED sort of fellow, not usually prone to fits of pique, but this morning something happened which induced in me a wobbler of outrageous proportions.

Last week, I had found myself completing a four page, A4-sized questionnaire to obtain, from Social Services, a piece of equipment for a patient.

What do you imagine it was that required such exhaustive documentation?

A dialysis machine, or perhaps his own personal MRI scanner?

No: a walking stick.

The saga started when Mr Haversham came to see me complaining about the pain in his hip. After nearly 50 years' hard graft on building sites around the north of England, he's developed a weather-beaten face, a colourful argot and a nasty dose of arthritis. He'll need a titanium replacement eventually, but for now he can get by with some anti-inflammatories and a stick. So I phoned Social Services and spoke to one of their gormless staff members to request just such an item.

The following day, the postman delivered the form for me to complete.

I considered this carefully, pondering questions such as, 'What is the client's view of the problem and preferred solution?' (his hip is knackered, he needs a stick but he would probably prefer a Lear Jet if there's one going), and 'Any risk of abuse or self-harm?' (I suppose in theory he could whack himself over the head with it). Then I scrawled across the form, 'He just needs a bloody walking stick.'

Today, one week later, I received a fresh form, together with a bossy memo upbraiding me for failing to fill in the original correctly.

But what *really* did it was that the envelope also contained *another* form, with a range of supplementary and entirely redundant questions, such as, 'Will the consumer require an Urdu interpreter?' (his name is *Haversham*, you morons) and 'Does the consumer require a full needs assessment?' (No, he needs, or 'requires' if you'd prefer, a *stick*.)

In a blind rage, I immediately phoned Social Services.

'Can I speak to someone in the walking stick department, please?' I said, and waited while the telephonist put me through. 'Right, it's Dr Copperfield from Bleak House surgery here,' I said. 'I have a patient who is 64 years old, he's got a lot of pain in his hip, I just want to order him a walking stick and...'

'You mean a personal mobility aid?'

'No, I mean a walking stick. I want to order my patient a walking stick to help alleviate his pain, and you buggers keep demanding that I fill in an ever-expanding series of forms just so he can get one. I'm his doctor, I say he needs it, it shouldn't need anything more than that.'

'Well, I'm afraid we have our procedures.'

'Stuff your bloody procedures! This man's in pain, he's worked all his life, he's paid his tax, he'd just like the possibility of being able to walk around a little more easily and now...'

'Please don't shout at me, or else I'll have to call my supervisor.'

Had I been in possession of the aforementioned stick at that moment, and had that employee of Social Services been in my presence, then I would have enjoyed nothing more than to have employed it as an impromptu anal dilator.

This type of scenario isn't unusual. Whether or not a patient will benefit from the largesse of the social services department seems to depend entirely upon how good the GP is at fabricating information and the mood of the person who receives the letter/form/phone call.

How far can the patient walk? Can the patient make himself a cup of tea? Does the patient likes sprouts? What football team does the patient support?

How the bloody hell do I know? Why don't they try asking the patient?

Needless to say, Mr Haversham is still waiting for his walking stick.

CARE PATHWAYS

'TOP OF THE morning to you, doctor,' said our resident Irish stereotype Mrs Peggotty as I breezed into work today. 'I've just put your post in your pigeonhole there. One of them got opened by mistake, I'm sorry. It's nothing personal – just something from the Department of Health or the PCT. I believe it's to do with these Care Pathways. Or is it one of those Model of Care things?'

She bustled off. I stopped breezing and began quietly simmering.

I walked to my pigeon hole and, sure enough, among the envelopes was a sheet headed 'Model of Care (COPD)'. I headed to my room, and once there I quickly moved to a good rolling boil.

You'd think there would never be any document more shredworthy than one headed 'Guidelines for GPs', but general practice is a place of a myriad marvels, and one of these is its infinite capacity to enrage us. Which explains the existence of 'Care Pathways'.

This new, appalling form of junk mail apparently 'depicts the patient's experience of his/her journey through the NHS process'. If that sounds like rubbish, that's because it is.

This week's involved Chronic Obstructive Pulmonary Disorder – a catch-all term used to describe a number of long-term breathing problems including chronic bronchitis and emphysema.

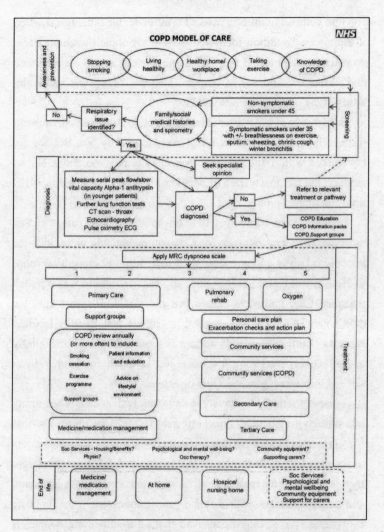

We get sent stacks of this stuff, it's all nonsense and this particular one was a classic of the type: impenetrable, meaningless, jargonistic drivel.

Even if you're the sort of sad, hopeless case who enjoys (and needs) flow charts like this, what bloody good is it as a decision aid? Where does it start? Where does it end? What happens if, for instance, you find yourself in the box marked 'Yes' under the other box marked 'Respiratory Condition Identified'? You have three possible exits – do you take them all? If not, which one *do* you take? It's a complete dog's breakfast and, try as I might, I simply cannot get inside the heads of the people who designed it.

It may seem trivial – after all, within around 30 seconds of opening the envelope, the sheet was lying crumpled in my bin. But we get bombarded with it and its sheer frequency grinds you down. Not to mention the fact that a team of people somewhere are spending NHS time and money producing it.

I could design a few myself, and it might be quite cathartic. For example, my Care Pathway for a patient demanding antibiotics for his cold involves a single step: an arrow from my consulting room to Hell. But the real point is this: 10 years ago, there was no such thing as 'Care Pathways'. Does that mean that, 10 years ago, we didn't care? Or is this just another fatuous and trendily-labelled exercise pointlessly complicating a process GPs have been quietly and effectively managing for years, just so that some poor sod can tick off the correct box in a DoH directive?

I fear it's actually much worse than that. Patient care is becoming increasingly fragmented: once, referral to a urologist meant just that – you referred the patient to a urologist. Now, before the patient gets to see the clever doctor with the white coat and superior expression, there's a pre-clinic assessment, a one-stop Prostates-R-Us shop, and an appointment with a nurse practitioner, purely to duplicate everything I've already done. And that's for something simple. If you're a newly-diagnosed diabetic, God help you, seriously. Your Care Pathway could take you right round the world, with prolonged stop-overs at chiropody, ophthalmology, endocrinology, cardiology risk assessment and smoking cessation, with an extra luggage allowance required for all your drugs.

This means that nowadays, when I refer patients, I no longer have the foggiest what will happen. I'm aware it will involve various stages and many appointments, but with whom, and when, and why, I really don't know.

The Care Pathway is supposed to resolve this problem. But, far from clarifying, it serves only to further obfuscate. It's written proof that no one has a clue what the hell is really going on.

Patients will be cared to death, or utterly neglected. They will become lost in the system, or caught in an infinite, nightmarish loop. Their only escape is to go through the door marked 'GP', which, oddly, is where they started – because they know that, while we may lead them off the Care Pathway, at least they'll be back on the straight and narrow.

No word of a lie, by the way: the second piece of post I opened this morning was a letter from the PCT informing me that dieticians, health visitors and the like had been commanded not to order any more stationery until the end of the financial year as a cost-saving measure.

THE FURTHER ADVENTURES OF MR NICKLEBY

'I'VE STILL GOT that buzzing in my ear.'

'Is that so, Mr Nickleby?'

'Yes, it bloody is. And the dizziness. And backache. And those spots in front of my eyes. And that bloating. I wondered if it was my thyroid.'

Deep breath. Calm. I heard myself saying, 'What made you think that?'

'One of my friends is a first aider, and he reckons I'm showing signs of an underactive thyroid. Or was it an overactive one? A wonky one, anyway.'

At this point, I should perhaps make clear that some time ago, when the practice was less familiar with Mr Nickleby, we took all his symptoms seriously. As a result, he has been questioned, prodded, tested and treated by a great variety of GPs, and then by a great variety of specialists, all of whom came to the same conclusion: there appeared to be nothing whatsoever wrong with him. And when he'd driven another partner or registrar to breaking point, the whole cycle would start all over again.

But, clearly, the combined forces of years of pontification and investigation by the most prestigious medical brains Clareshire has to offer are nothing compared to the wisdom of a first aider.

'Mr Nickleby,' I said, as I handed over the form, white-flag stylee, 'You shall have your thyroid test. But if it's in any way abnormal, I'll eat my own head.'

SNIP SNIP

I LIKE TO play a little guessing game with myself where I try to work out why a patient is here before he or she opens his or her mouth. It helps me to avoid being driven bonkers by the viral and emotional sniffles of the average surgery.

So: elderly man hobbling in with sore foot in a slipper? Gout.

Two teenage girls, one of whom says, 'Go on...' while the other stares at her feet? Morning-after pill.

Try this one from the other day: a determined-looking woman, all but dragging a blushing, sheepish man behind her?

No idea?

Here's a clue: he's protecting his gonads in the manner of a defender facing a Ronaldo free kick.

It was Mr and Mrs Meagles, and her opening gambit was, 'He needs the snip, doctor.'

Bingo! If only I was as good with the lottery numbers.

'He's not keen, but I've told him it's that or no more... you know. Only, we've already got five kids and I couldn't cope with any more.'

I looked at the great inseminator, who was studiously examining the pale brown nylon carpet.

'How do you feel about this, Mr Meagles?' I said.

'He doesn't want it, but I've told him he's having it and that's all there is to it,' said his wife. 'Ignore him.'

'Someone said he'd heard it was like having it cut off,' said her husband, meeting my gaze temporarily, before developing a keen interest in the wall above my head.

Bloody Richard Madeley. A while back he apparently said on some chat show or other that the pain from his vasectomy felt more like the doctors had chopped rather than snipped. Ever since then, men 'requesting' the same procedure will attend the surgery only if dragged there by the short and curlies.

By implying that this simple operation could leave the average bloke an unwilling member of the No Member Club, Madeley gave men an excuse they really don't need. They already had a long list of objections to trot out to dodge the scalpel – such as the concern that it might increase the risk of heart disease and prostate or testicle cancer.

Wrong, wrong and wrong. In fact, there is some evidence that vasectomised men actually live longer than average, though this probably reflects the detrimental effect of having any more than 2.4 children swarming around you, rather than any magical benefits of the snip.

'Look,' I said, 'there's nothing to it. After a week or so, you'll forget it was ever done.'

He met my eyes again. 'I just don't like the idea of it,' he said.

'Who would?' I said. 'Any man who *does* like the idea of cold steel meeting warm scrotum needs a psychiatrist, not a surgeon. But grow up and stop whining and think about someone else for a change. Your wife's done her bit – give her a break.'

'I *told* you,' said Mrs Meagles, with a note of triumph in her voice and a glint of fire in her eye. 'You listen to doctor Copperfield, if you know what's good for you.'

I was warming to her by the second.

'But what about… you know… will it affect whether I…'

'For God's sake man,' I hissed. 'We're all adults. You mean will it affect your sex life? Yes, it will – for the better.'

Which is true. What you lose in fertility you gain in spontaneity and safety. You can say goodbye to flailing around in the dark, not knowing whether you've grabbed a pack of condoms or your contact lenses, and you can stop panicking that an *in flagrante* attack of cramp in your partner is a pill-induced DVT.

'Look,' he said, with a sidelong glance at his wife. 'How about if I just have one side done, just to see how it goes?'

I sighed, and began tapping on my keyboard. For some reason, men don't seem to have any of these problems requesting a vasectomy reversal. From a psychodynamic perspective, that's probably because they see this as a restoration of machismo rather than a form of castration. Which is why, when they walk in with their new partner to request unvasectomising, they look pretty confident and relaxed.

Or maybe it's just that they know it's not actually available on the NHS.

ANOTHER BLOODY MEETING

TUESDAY MORNINGS AT the pebble-dashed pillbox that is our branch surgery are never much fun.

Firstly, I'm often the only doctor there and as well as looking after my own cases I get to provide second opinions for the nurse and to sign all her prescriptions.

Judging by the number of antibiotics she doles out she's a major shareholder in several pharmaceutical companies. I don't have time to query them, I just sign 'em and send the happy punters on their way.

A few skirmishes with the ASBO-toting crowd from the Staffordshire Cross estate and a couple of lunatic visit requests from the local nursing home set me right up for our Tuesday lunchtime staff meeting back at Bleak House. I arrived with enough time to spare to take a much-needed leak, grab a sandwich and wash my hands, not necessarily in that order. I certainly didn't have time to check my pigeon hole for messages, urgent or otherwise.

I dashed from the surgery door to the loo and, via a brief encounter with the wash basin and hand dryer, into the coffee room to find out which sandwiches the gannets had turned their noses up at. A grated yellow cheese and tomato sandwich ('Reduced'), a prawn mayonnaise baguette that I knew from previous encounters would reset the bar as far as slime-based snack products were concerned and a plastic package containing a selection of tired lettuce leaves were on offer.

It's not like this on fucking Peak Practice, I thought to myself. *I've been grafting like a navvy and I get to eat crap whilst listening to some berk from Berk Central prattle on about...*

Which reminded me, I had no idea what today's meeting was about. Or who was presenting it. If it was my turn to lead off, it was going to be a disaster.

I glanced up at the Big Board to check the week's timetable. Out of the corner of my eye I caught sight of the 'Recent Deaths' section: two B-list Hollywood actors, a Russian ballet dancer, a Portuguese poet and a familiar name.

Rebecca Bagnet.

RASH HOUR

ROUGHLY HALF OF the patients I saw yesterday were young children with sniffles, dragged along to surgery by their worried mums.

I'd known it would be like this since seeing the front page of the local paper at the petrol station on my way in to work that morning.

MENINGITIS HITS TOWN, it yelled, and I didn't need to be Nostradamus to predict that everything would immediately go into meltdown – it always does after that sort of headline. The phone lines go bananas and GPs and casualty doctors are confronted with florid descriptions of children who are consistently 'at death's door', dramatically failing to 'keep anything down' and invariably 'burning up'.

It was all depressingly familiar: welcome to the meningitis season!

Considering that any individual's chances of getting bacterial meningitis are pretty remote, an astonishing number of out-of-hours phone calls and emergency consultations result from mothers and fathers with the dread fear that their kid might be the next victim.

By now, most people are surely aware of the 'classic' symptoms of meningococcal infection: the unholy triad of neck stiffness, a dislike of bright lights and a blotchy red rash which doesn't fade when a glass is rolled over it. After all, every winter, well-meaning charities publish millions of leaflets advising parents and teachers what to look out for and when to seek help if they think a child is ill.

Unfortunately, these textbook diagnostic clues are not the whole story. For starters, they tend to affect teenagers and older children, rather than toddlers. Plus, they don't always all show up, and when they do it's often not until the disease is in its later stages, when it can be too late: within two or three hours of the tell-tale rash appearing, for instance, it's entirely possible that a hospital paediatrician will be in the Sister's office breaking bad news to sobbing parents and offering them tea and sympathy. I have been there, done that and have the T-shirt: it's a terrible thing, trust me.

The 'stiff neck, rash and photophobia' mantra is so ingrained into our minds that even GPs – many of whom have never seen a child with meningitis outside hospital – can quite easily dismiss the diagnosis in error purely because one or more of those symptoms is absent.

But that's not the worst part. The truth is that meningitis usually kicks off with 'non specific' symptoms like fever and vomiting. Unfortunately, just about every childhood infection starts exactly same way. And – contrary to public belief – there is no magic meningitisometer available to us by which we can distinguish, at this early stage, between a simple virus and something rather more catastrophic. So you can imagine the fun we have in the middle of a flu epidemic. We can't send every feverish child up to hospital – it's overloaded as it is. All we can do is hope mum remembers our advice to contact us again if junior gets worse, and accept that someone, somewhere is going to have to take the 'My baby had meningitis and the GP said it was just a virus' headline on the chin.

Over my career, I've seen four cases – as far as I know – and none of them had a rash.

I admitted three of them after the first visit, which puts me slightly ahead of the game, and they all made complete recoveries.

I only caught a glimpse of the fourth, who just happened to be playing quietly in the corner of the bedroom while I examined her elder brother. She died in her sleep the next night. Awful.

Each of my three survivors had a subtle early warning symptom that had me worried enough to send them in to hospital. One had freezing cold hands and feet despite a high fever, another looked pale and was unable to stand without help, the third had a blueish tinge to his lips and a slightly bulging fontanelle, the soft spot where the skull bones join together just above the forehead. These symptoms are pretty vague, but any doctor worth his or her salt will take them seriously.

My three patients all looked sick enough to need admitting to hospital and they all got a potentially life-saving antibiotic injection while we waited for the ambulance to arrive. As a result, my credibility with the local hospital's children's ward was assured. For a time, local graffiti artists modified their handiwork to read 'Copperfield is God' – a nice change from the usual 'knobhead' stuff – and eminent paediatricians would seek me out at post-graduate meetings to congratulate me on my astute clinical acumen.

Fourteen years later, the kid who'd had the freezing cold hands broke into my car and nicked my CD player.

COMMUNICATION PROBLEMS

MEDICINE IS ALL about doctor-patient communication, according to the experts.

Mind you, these are 'experts' who run 'consultation skills workshops' at which one usually learns nothing except that anyone who uses the word 'workshop' without reference to light engineering is to be avoided.

The fact is that doctor-patient communication is not the whole story, or even the biggest part of it, as the little drama of Barry and Sharon Varden showed.

'Doc,' said Barry the other week. 'It's the wife. She's seeing double.'

'Hmmm?' I said. Most people who say they're seeing double, aren't, they're just dizzy. 'Are you sure?'

'Yes, I'm absolutely sure,' he said. 'She can see two of me and she ain't sure which one to slap. Plus she keeps falling over. And them tablets the other doctor gave her ain't helped, neither.'

I arranged for her to have her blood tested and started digging. What I uncovered was... interesting.

Sharon suffers from epilepsy, and her condition is difficult to control.

Until recently she took a 200mg dose of an anticonvulsant drug, carbamazepine, twice a day.

Her neurologist wrote to us asking that her dose be doubled, so we rewrote her repeat prescription to issue a 400mg tablet, twice daily.

The following week she saw a general physician at the same hospital.

He told her to take *three* tablets a day, rather than two.

Now, either he wanted her to move from 800mg to 1200mg, just after she'd been bounced up from 400mg (most unlikely, as raising anticonvulsant doses needs to be done very carefully indeed), or he wasn't aware that the tablets had changed.

I suspect the latter: he *assumed* she still had 200mg tablets at home, not 400mg, and *thought* he was raising her to 600mg.

But assumption is the mother of all screw-ups. In fact, she'd already picked up a month's supply of the double strength version, something she unfortunately neglected to mention to him; this meant he was actually trebling her dose in a matter of days.

Why he wasn't aware of the earlier change in dosage, I'm not sure. Maybe he didn't have the neurologist's notes. Maybe he did, but mis-read them. Maybe he only looked at Sharon's medical clinic notes and not the neurology notes, thinking they weren't relevant.

Whatever, this was quite dramatic, to say the least. As I say, anticonvulsants are dangerous things: too little and they don't work, too much and we're talking toxicity. I usually ask patients to increase their daily carbamazepine dose by 200mg every Monday until they start to throw up or fall over. Then they go back to whatever dose they were taking the previous Monday and have a blood level estimated a few days later.

Luckily, despite the sudden ramping up of her dosage, Sharon was still with us and at least things couldn't get worse – at least, not until a psychiatrist showed up and decided she needed an antidepressant to cheer her up and, hey, it might even help her worsening giddiness.

He gave her fluoxetine, better known as Prozac.

And that was the cock-up that broke the camel's back – if you'll pardon a mixed metaphor.

Carbamazepine, like most other drugs we prescribe, is broken down as it passes through the liver. Unfortunately, Prozac is broken down by the same enzyme system. So while the liver is busily dealing with the Prozac that Sharon's just necked, more of the carbamazepine gets through unscathed. Net effect, another unintentional increase in Sharon's already excessive dose. (Unintentional but entirely predictable, if only Dr Freud had been bothered to check the 'Interactions' section of his drug textbook. Most doctors know that every other drug in the world interferes with carbamazepine, so before handing over a prescription to a patient taking it we consult the *British National Formulary*. It's there on page 642 of the current edition: 'Plasma concentration of carbamazepine – increased by fluoxetine.' In layman's terms, 'plasma concentration' is the amount of the drug floating around in the bloodstream where it can do what it does.)

No wonder Sharon couldn't see straight: the lab tests I ordered showed that her plasma carbamazepine level was four times the ideal. She stopped taking the drug for a few days and her double vision, dizziness and loss of balance evaporated.

So what's my point?

Communication breakdown about dose increase somewhere between neurologist and physician; then psychiatrist didn't think about the carbamazepine/fluoxetine conflict. No one, apart from the neurologist, told her GP – me – anything.

Except Barry, that is, who told me that his wife really was seeing double.

Whatever the workshop people say, it's when doctor-*doctor* communication slips up that things really kick off.

FUNNY TURNS

THE FIRST LETTER I opened in my morning post the other day was from a consultant dermatologist to whom I had referred a hatchet-faced old boot called Mrs Rudge.

'Dear Tony,' it began. 'Thank you for asking my opinion regarding this delightful lady's…'

I put the letter down, rubbed my eyes and re-read that opening sentence. Delightful lady? Mrs Rudge?

Then I remembered: it was a private referral (the 'Dear Tony' should have provided a clue). Mrs Rudge may indeed be 'delightful' in the sense that she has a valid Mastercard with a five-figure credit limit, but for an honest description I refer you to *my* opening line, above.

At least if she ever demands to see the letter, it will be clear that the obsequious consultant knows upon which side his bread is buttered.

Because you do know that you now have the right to receive copies of letters that your GP and consultant have exchanged about you, right?

That doesn't mean it's a good idea to ask. Most of them will consist of educated guesses about diagnostic possibilities, the results of any ongoing investigations and the odd bit of banter. Mine might begin: 'Dear Simon, I thought I'd waft this kiddie past you and see if your paediatrician's syndrome detector twitches…'

Letters about undescended testicles will invariably include the clause, 'spot the ball', or an oblique Peter Cook reference: 'I have absolutely nothing against this young chap's right testis; the problem is, neither has he.'

So, yes, doctors' letters can be fun. But, be warned, don't read any unless you can cope with finding the words 'multiple sclerosis' somewhere in one about you.

Everybody, but everybody, has a letter in their file that contains the abbreviation 'MS'. It's the inevitable result of telling a doctor about any episode that involved dizziness, numbness or double vision.

When I was in my twenties, I developed a painful burning sensation down my left thigh. I was convinced I'd finish my studies in a wheelchair. I have never seen my medical record, but I'll wager there's a letter in there reading: 'Narcissistic med student plonker with trapped nerve. Jeans two sizes too small. Thinks he has MS. Advised look up meralgia paraesthetica in textbooks and buy baggier trousers.'

If there isn't, there should be.

You, too, will have a funny turn one day. Whether it's a midsummer faint or a low blood sugar incident after skipping breakfast, it will probably be trivial but your GP will record it. The first thing to figure out about fits 'n' faints is which diagnostic basket to put them into. There's one labelled: 'Funny turns – cardiac' and others called 'neurological', 'diabetic' and 'miscellaneous'.

Assuming that your pulse is regular and you're not an obvious drunk, he will write: 'Funny turn – ?epilepsy ?diabetes ?MS' (the question marks meaning 'possible'). If you need a specialist opinion, the same list of possibilities will appear in your referral letter to confirm that they have been considered.

This will put the wind right up the 99 per cent of you whose dizzy spells prove to be benign, but the alternative is that doctors' letters will turn into bland shadows of their former selves and become virtually worthless. If I don't mention possible diagnoses in my letters, some consultants will assume that I can't think of any. Eventually, when a diagnosis is made, patients will assume that I hadn't even considered it, when, in truth, I was hoping to spare them unnecessary anxiety.

BACKACHE

'I PUT MY BACK out last night, Doc,' said Mick Warden. 'I was just bending down to stick something in the dishwasher and – bam! I couldn't straighten back up again. It's bloody agony.'

Over half of us will suffer at least one severe attack of backache in our lives, and more than a million people in the UK say they are 'disabled' by it. GP consultations for 'lumbago' cost the NHS £140 million a year, and when you add in physiotherapy, hospital treatment and prescriptions, the annual back-pain bill runs to £1.6 billion.

Mick's 25. He plays pub football in the winter, village cricket in the summer and rides a bike to the gym once a week. He's pretty fit. But I didn't doubt he was suffering: you could see from the way he stood, wincing, as he spoke, that his pain was genuine.

I got him to try and touch his toes, then try to straighten up. I laid him down on the exam couch, lifted his left leg into the air and heard a barely-stifled rude word as he felt what seemed like an electric shock go along his sciatic nerve all the way down to his toes.

As I did so, my mind wandered to some interesting research from the USA. This suggests that in the majority of cases like this there is actually no anatomical abnormality to be found – no slipped disc, no torn ligament – and that a patient's likelihood of developing back pain therefore has as much to do with his mind as his spine. One hundred volunteers had fluid injected into the area around their spinal discs. The theory was, this procedure would cause discomfort to those who were actually going to go on and develop back problems. During a four-year follow-up, some subjects indeed went on to get backache. The weird thing was, they weren't the predicted ones with wonky spines – or the ones with a positive 'ceiling sign' (i.e., inject fluid, patient hits roof). The only valuable predictive test was a psychological assessment: those with 'coping skills' were not likely to complain about back pain; those without them were.

Back to Mick. The fact is, whatever I do – or don't do – for people like him, they are almost guaranteed to make a full recovery in a few weeks. The best I can realistically offer is to ease their symptoms during that time with injections, pills and embrocations.

After a brief explanation of the diagnosis, a dollop of arm-around-the-shoulder sympathy and a prescription for an anti-inflammatory painkiller, I told him to take a few days off work, let his wife load the dishwasher and – most important of all – keep as mobile as he could.

He looked a bit doubtful. 'Aren't you going to send me for some tests or something?' he said.

'I don't think that will be necessary,' I said.

A fit young bloke with occasional back trouble like Mick shouldn't be troubling his local orthopaedic surgeon or going for barrages of tests – and luckily, he didn't have private medical insurance. If he had, he'd have been put through a series of increasingly unpleasant investigations before being given a clean bill of health – an expensive way of saying, 'It's all in your mind.'

CARING FOR OLD FOLKS

IF THERE'S ONE thing which cheers me up, it's hearing that Sami Patel has gone out to see an old lady at Rosemount Gardens Retirement Home.

Sami is a Nicole Farhi / iPhone / Oakleys sort of chap: delving into the contents of Mrs Whimple's bedpan is very much *not* his style. In fact, it's just about the only thing guaranteed to wipe the smile off his insufferably smug face.

He was out at Rosemount at the crack of dawn the other morning, and as a result I found myself spending the day grinning inanely, humming *Ode To Joy* and being unexpectedly pleasant to the patients.

I once worked as a junior doctor in a psychiatric hospital. My empire consisted of two wards and my job description, though unwritten, was clear. I was expected to keep the acute ward full, locking the door behind me to prevent an exodus of the insane on to the streets. I was also expected to do my bit to empty the geriatric ward earmarked for closure in the 'medium-term'. No heroic resuscitation efforts, Copperfield, thanks.

Then someone realised that a lot of these bed-blockers could be dumped into suburbia – under the noble cover of 'Care in the Community' – to free up funds for more deserving causes, like paying NHS managers exorbitant salaries to oversee the development of baffling flow charts, and providing them with gold-plated pensions.

Nowadays, no market town is complete without its purpose-built granny-stacker, boasting ample parking for visiting families, a teasing view of the local cemetery and a weekly visit from a semi-retired crooner to lead a sing-along.

These magnolia-decorated twilight zones are divided into separate units catering for the sane and mobile (residential), the sane but immobile (nursing), the confused and *too* mobile (elderly mentally ill – residential) and the demented and thankfully immobile (elderly mentally ill – nursing).

Rosemount is a privately-run nursing home (broadly sane but relatively chairbound) operated by a group which runs half a dozen or more such places, and every Monday and Thursday evening after surgery, you'll see my little blue Nissan hatchback parked in the 'Ambulances Only' bay outside.

Actually, I quite like looking after the elderly residents – I like the way they accept their physical limitations, and how they offer to buy their paracetamol from Asda to save the NHS some money. But the ward rounds are torture.

Every now and again, a newly-appointed nurse tells me that 'Mrs Podsnap's urine smells funny, doctor', and expects an answer that doesn't take the piss. After a few months they get up to speed: 'Mrs Podsnap has a low-grade fever and complains of pain passing urine, doctor. The urine tested positive for blood and nitrites. I've sent a specimen to the lab for a confirmatory culture but in the meantime should we start treating her presumed bladder infection?'

Similar learning curves are scaled about Mrs Podsnap's cough, her leg ulcer, her piles and her painful hip.

Unfortunately, after this brief respite of relative sanity, I will arrive one day to be greeted by a complete stranger, and the whole whirligig will begin again: 'Good evening, doctor. Mrs Podsnap's urine smells funny.'

The problem is that, after a few weeks in the job, the decent nurses are either labelled 'team leaders', and moved to a failing home elsewhere in the group, or they leave to join a locum agency so that they can earn reasonable money. I often feel like suggesting to the group managers that they study the poster in the dry cleaner's window across the road: 'We work up to a standard, not down to a price.'

I'd have a word with the people who designed the last GP contract, too. This makes it clear that the essence of medical care for the elderly is not – as I believe it should be – to ensure that they are warm, well-fed and as symptom-free as possible. From now on, it's to lower aggressively their cholesterol levels, confiscate their sherry, nag them about their 30-a-day (and 60-year) smoking habit and ferry them to utterly pointless smoking cessation clinics every six months until they eventually die, thoroughly miserable and utterly bewildered.

ONE HUNDRED, NOT OUT

'AH, BLESS,' said Dr Emma in the common room today, wrinkling her nose and smiling. 'Ah… that's lovely, that is.'

Restraining the urge to upchuck my lunch, I looked up to see her scribbling on something and handing it back to an expectant Mrs Peggotty. The receptionist advanced towards me.

'Now then, Dr Copperfield,' she said. 'Will you sign this card, please? It's for Mrs Sikes.'

'Mrs Sikes?' I said, blankly.

'Yes, Mrs Sikes,' said Mrs Peggotty. 'Only, she's a hundred years old next week, so I thought we'd send her a little something from the practice.'

Out of the corner of my eye I saw Sami Patel – never comfortable around the elderly – cram the remnants of his lunchtime sandwich into his mouth and slink from the room.

'Do we have to?' I said. 'I mean, *why*? It's not as if we want to encourage people to reach that sort of age. Is it?'

'If it's good enough for the Queen,' said Mrs Peggotty, firmly, 'it's good enough for the likes of you. Sign here.'

Meekly, though slightly under protest, I did as I was told.

I have to admit, there is something special about the number 100 – the 100 metres is the most glamorous event at the Olympics, the cricketer raises his bat to mark his century and, as Mrs Peggotty pointed out, Liz will send you a telegram to mark you reaching your own personal ton.

I'm not against any of that; I'm just not sure that doctors should get into the same game.

Some years ago, insightfully I felt, one GP suggested that Her Majesty's congratulatory telegrams ought instead to go to the centenarian's family doctors. If the Queen ever takes up this bright idea, I hope she also includes a few words giving the medics permission to – how can I put this gently? – 'soft pedal' a bit from then on. If the task fell instead to the GP's local Primary Care Trust then a similar sentiment might be expressed less diplomatically: 'Oi! Copperfield! Re Mrs Aida Gaspard, born May 6, 1910. Here's your Employee of the Bloody Month Award and now could you please pack it in? Do you think we're made of money?'

Put bluntly, old people are expensive to run.

Billions are spent on interventions that are often inappropriate for elderly patients, whose health imperatives really don't include getting their cholesterol level below 5mmol/l. Snooker-loopy geriatricians amuse themselves by giving every patient a red pill, a brown pill, a yellow pill and so on all the way up to the black, at huge cost and not much benefit: most independent old people are smart enough to leave most of their prescribed drugs in the boxes and just take the pink ones that stop their joints from aching.

The trouble starts after they move into a residential home like the Rosemount, when Matron takes charge and makes *sure* that they take all seven of their prescribed tablets at 8 o'clock sharp. The consequences are entirely predictable: it's like a game of medical Buckaroo, where you hang as many different medications on to Grandma's prescription chart as you can and eventually a clinically important drug interaction kicks in and the whole thing takes off.

It's taxing enough when two or three new old folks are admitted to the Rosemount, but I was chatting to an old friend in another practice in a town a dozen or so miles away yesterday and she informed me that she was about to confront the nightmare scenario. A new home was just about to open next door to her surgery, which will see her dealing with 50 or 60 new residents in a single week, each with prescription charts that run to six or seven pages.

'It's going to make spinning plates at a circus look like child's play,' she groaned. For once, I had some sympathy. I could picture the scene: as quickly as they settle in at one end of the corridor, they start dropping like ninepins at the other, succumbing to the effects of unaccustomed doses of blood-pressure reducers, sedating analgesics and antidepressants. Ambulances ferrying them to the local hospital would be fighting for space in the car park with mini-cabs delivering more potential victims with their families and suitcases. Somewhere near the eye of the storm I could just about make out my friend contemplating her early retirement.

Sir Richard Doll, who died recently at the age of 92, famously demonstrated the link between cigarette smoking and lung cancer. He worked well beyond retirement age but courted controversy when he told pensioners not to expect NHS time and money to be spent on research into prolonging life and advised them instead to 'live dangerously'.

And you know what? He was spot on. So wake up and smell the Horlicks. I simply refuse to believe that all those nonagenarians enjoy watching *Loose Women* or *The All New Scooby Doo Show* in their communal lounges every Monday afternoon, so let's see them on Saga outings, bungee-jumping their way to the end of a long innings.

WHAT ARE THE ODDS?

ON MY WAY home at night, I drive along an arterial road linking us to the metropolis.

Every now and then, you'll see cellophane bunches of flowers and rain-sodden teddies fastened to a lamppost, but now there's a new distraction – a sign detailing the number of injuries suffered along that particular stretch in the previous year.

It warns: '68 casualties in 2009'.

I can't be the only person who drives past by thinking that those aren't bad odds. I'm no expert in traffic, but I reckon several million vehicles a year use the road: 68 injuries isn't all that bad.

There are similar signs along the roads running out of Manchester to the south through Moss Side – '56 injured in 2009' – but last time I was there I saw that someone, with typical northern directness, had appended a supplementary hand-painted note: 'And ten of them were drive bys'.

The warning is clear – drive down here and you take your chances.

Everyone knows that life is a crap shoot from cradle to grave (even if they don't know what a crap shoot is). This message was lost, though, on the bloke from the Royal College of GPs I heard on Radio 5 Live the other day telling listeners that GPs are failing 'patients who have gambling problems'.

I'll bet you can guess what came next: we 'must do more' for these people (also known as 'losers' – no-one who *wins* on the horses sees it as a problem, do they?).

A compulsive gambler told the BBC that he'd gone to his GP shaking and depressed because he was utterly skint, hoping that, and I quote verbatim, 'they might have an inkling as to what was going on'.

Of course, we GPs are famous for our clairvoyant skills. We know that out of an entire morning surgery only one or two patients will present with problems that actually need our help. We know any e-mail from the PCT marked 'High Priority' will be dross, and so can be deleted immediately. We know that the new drugs are unlikely to be any better than the old ones.

But even though we possess astonishing powers of prediction we augment them with a bit of voodoo known as 'Recording the History of the Presenting Complaint'.

Put simply, we ask the patient what is wrong. In this case, it would have been: 'I'm depressed because they've repossessed my BMW.'

Then, brilliantly, we ask them what they think the reason might be for this occurrence.

This is the patient's chance to fess up that their infallible system to break the bank at Monte Carlo wasn't infallible after all, that a tip on a 33-1 outsider at Kempton Park isn't usually a safe bet and that the Lotto has turned out to be nothing but a devious form of indirect taxation on the poor, stupid and greedy.

But like all addicts covering their tracks, they'll lie. There's always an excuse. A cash flow problem, hassle from the VAT man or the Inland Revenue.

It's always somebody else's fault – you can put money on that.

WHAT MR NICKLEBY DID NEXT

'I'VE STILL GOT that buzzing in my ear.'

Ah, but at least my head is safe. His thyroid test has come back normal. *Quelle surprise.*

'So what *is* causing all my symptoms, then?'

I looked him in the eye. It struck me that I had three options.

One: I could murder him. I thought about this, just for a moment, then rejected it. Not a good career move.

Two: I could run screaming from the room. This was a more realistic possibility, and potentially quite cathartic. I took a little longer to file it under 'abort'.

It had to be Option Three.

'Mr Nickleby. I've taken the opportunity to have a really good look back through all your records. I've gone through all the opinions, the tests, the treatment. And I do believe…' I leaned in closer, and, in an effort to exude authority and solemnity, I put down my pen and thoughtfully stroked my chin. 'I do believe, Mr Nickleby, that I finally know what's wrong with you.'

He didn't know whether to be alarmed or relieved. But he was certainly interested. 'You do? You know what's wrong with me?'

'I do. I do know what's wrong with you.'

He actually became quite excited. 'Well, what is it, then, doctor?'

'You have something called…' I paused so he got the full effect. 'Somatisation disorder.'

190

'I do? I have somatisation disorder?' He savoured the words. 'Somatisation disorder... I knew it... I knew there was something wrong!'

'Indeed,' I repeated. 'Somatisation disorder.'

'Ha!' he said. I'd never seen him look so cheerful. 'And all those other doctors – they all said it was in my mind! I knew it. All in my mind! So tell me, what exactly is this "somatisation disorder"?'

At that point, I started to panic slightly. Somatisation disorder = physical symptoms with a psychological basis. Not, note, malingering. The symptoms are genuine: the dry mouth and racing heart caused by the nerves of giving a best man's speech are real, but they're not caused by any physical disease. The problems really arise when the individual can't make the link between the psyche and the soma, and therefore remains convinced that there is something 'organically' wrong – a state which increases the tension and so may exacerbate the symptoms. It's very difficult to manage. One of the GP's key tasks is to protect the patient from hospitals and their attendant nasty tests and treatments. Another is to protect the hospitals from these patients.

I repeated his question, playing for time. 'So... *they* all said it was... in your mind? And now *you*... you want to know exactly what somatisation disorder is?'

At this point, almost involuntarily, I screwed up my eyes. I was reminded of an incident from my childhood when I spilt Ribena on my mum's new carpet. A reasonable strategy at the time seemed to be to shut my eyes and pray that God might magic it all away. I'm an atheist, and I suspect that, even then, I didn't really believe in God – but I was prepared to, especially if He was good with Ribena stains. Maybe, just maybe, when I opened my eyes, Mr Nickleby would have gone. Then I wouldn't have to explain that somatisation disorder, which had so gloriously usurped That Which All The Other Doctors Said Was In His Mind, meant that it was all in his mind.

'Dr Copperfield, are you OK?'

'Oh, just feeling a bit woozy.'

'OK, look doctor,' he said, genuinely concerned. 'Don't you worry. I'll book another appointment.'

And with that, he was gone.

HEART FAILURE

I MENTIONED HEART FAILURE earlier (it was one of the many illnesses suffered by Mr Endell, the elderly and distressed chap who suffered multiple inhumane frustrations at the hands of the hospital).

At least once a week, I find myself discussing this condition with a patient or relative and finding that they haven't a clue what it actually means.

Yesterday's contestant was Tom Traddles, who doubles as my trusty car mechanic. He was suffering from the classic symptoms: breathlessness on exercise, ankle swelling and profound tiredness.

'Heart failure?' he said. 'Yeah, that's when the coronary wotsit fails and the heart packs up, innit? And then you're brown bread, 'cos your heart's stopped.'

Not even close: congestive cardiac failure is not a synonym for cardiac arrest, the correct technical term for the situation Tom outlined; it is a medical condition in its own right and is the commonest reason for urgent hospital admission in the over 70s.

At medical school, I endured lectures about left heart failure, right heart failure, congestive cardiac failure, pure pump failure, low output heart failure, high output heart failure, third heart sounds, fourth heart sounds, HOCM (pronounced, amusingly, 'hokum'), COCM ('cokum'), cardiac asthma and something known as 'Cor Pulmonale', which I swear was the name of my great aunt Jessica's bungalow in Blackpool. To be fair, even I find it confusing, which may explain why apparently only three per cent of 'persons in the street' have much understanding.

Put very, very *Ladybird Book of Internal Medicine* simply, heart failure results from heart muscle damage caused by prolonged high blood pressure, a previous heart attack or, in very unlucky young folk, a virus. The damaged heart is unable to pump as efficiently as it should. During exercise it cannot increase the amount of blood delivered to working tissues, clear excess fluid from the lungs or pump it back up from parts of the body nearest to the ground, which, unless you're bed-ridden or a three-toed sloth, would usually be your ankles, hence the swelling.

A while back, the British Heart Foundation produced a graphic advertising campaign featuring an actor fighting for breath with his head in a polythene bag. If you ask anybody who's in a position to know, this is exactly how a cardiac failure patient with waterlogged lungs feels. Moronically, the Advertising Standards Authority pulled the ads because the images might encourage 'copycat' behaviour.

Heart failure, at least in the early stages, is treatable. Combination drug therapy reduces breathlessness, cuts limb-swelling and improves exercise tolerance. Once in a while, there's a treatable underlying cause such as an overactive thyroid gland, anaemia or an irregular heart rhythm. So if granny's puffed out halfway up the stairs, her pulse is racing and her ankles are the size of tree trunks, a visit to her GP might be a wise investment of half an hour of her time.

I wanted to get Tom into Outpatients quickly for an echocardiogram – an ultrasound test which determines how much blood the heart is pumping.

This is where my frustrations began. As we know, if he'd been suffering from a suspected cancer he would have been in within two weeks, whether he needed to be seen that quickly or not, in order that the government could issue press releases about cancer waiting times. But although congestive cardiac failure is in many ways more serious than a lot of cancers, Tom has zero hope of being seen within two weeks. In fact, I doubt I'll get an echo done on him within the next eight to ten weeks – valuable time when it comes to identifying and alleviating a pretty unpleasant condition, leaving him suffering needlessly in the interim. Scandalous? You may think so. I suspect the trouble is that cardiac failure is not a sexy topic, as it primarily affects people in the last few years of their lives. The Heath Secretary gets no brownie points for announcing schemes to combat it, and the do-gooders rattling tins outside Sainsbury's cannot compete with charities that fund research into conditions that make grown men go dewy-eyed, such as childhood leukaemia: they'll put their hand into their pocket for their little Princess, but not for their dear white-haired old mum.

Perhaps it's simply the use of the word 'failure' that needs addressing: let's change the name of the diagnosis to 'reduced cardiac success' and see if that makes any difference.

WHY MEN ARE BETTER THAN WOMEN AT DEALING WITH PAIN

'IT'S OFFICIAL,' I said. 'It says here that there *is* a difference between the sexes after all.'

We were waiting to begin our Monday meeting. I was flicking through the newspaper, Dr Emma was diligently reading the agenda and Sami Patel was filling his face with Hob Nobs (this is my third or fourth attempt at product placement – I hope McVitie's are reading).

'Tell me about it,' he said, spraying crumbs everywhere in the process. 'Women look terrible with moustaches, for a start.'

Dr Emma took a more mature line. 'What's the difference?' she said. 'Apart from the obvious?'

'According to this report by the Chronic Pain Policy Coalition, whoever they are, you lot feel pain more than we do and you cope with it less well, too.'

'Yeah,' said Sami. 'So let's have no more of that guff about women being designed to endure the pain of childbirth or that rubbish about man flu. Our pain is real, do you hear? Real.'

Dr Emma snorted and went back to the agenda. Sami grabbed another Hob Nob and I read on.

According to the coalition's spokeswoman, GPs haven't noticed that men and women behave differently – a statement so nonsensical that it actually gave me a headache.

There are at least a dozen important things that a patient can tell me about their pain. Getting these details from a man is like pulling teeth, but a woman can sit down and rattle them off without so much as a pause for breath. And I *have* noticed this difference.

Mrs Westlock can tell me where it hurts, when it hurts, what brings it on, what makes it worse, how long it lasts and what makes it better. These diagnostic nuggets whizz past so quickly that I barely have time to write them down.

But asking Mr Westlock to describe the pain he's in is a complete waste of time. He almost certainly won't have the vocabulary and I'll have to resort to putting words in his mouth: 'Would you say it was a sharp, stabbing pain or is it more like a dull ache? Does it build up and then fade away, or is it pretty constant? How about when you move; does that makes it worse or better?'

'I dunno Doc, but I'll tell you one thing ...' Here he will pause for effect, as though he were about to divulge the combination for the bullion vault at the Bank of England. 'It hurts like buggery.'

When faced with a bloke in pain it's usually better to ignore the words and check out his body language. Pointing to where it hurts with a single finger is manspeak for 'sharp and stabbing'. Waving the palm of the hand over the abdomen means 'stomach cramps' and clutching a fist over the chest means, 'It's not really indigestion and I should have dialled 999.'

Brain scans apparently show that when men are in pain – typically created by having their arm stuck in a bucket of iced water for an extended period – the area concerned with analysis and problem-solving is the most active. When women are subjected to the same painful stimulus it's the limbic system, the part of the brain concerned with emotional responses, that kicks into overdrive.

When men are asked to forget how annoyed they feel about being in pain and to focus more on the unpleasant sensation itself, their level of pain reduces. This doesn't happen in women; it's as if they can't divorce the emotional from the physical aspects of discomfort.

Consider these real world examples, two painful conditions with no apparent physical cause – fibromyalgia and irritable bowel syndrome. Both are much more common in women than men and don't get better if treated with standard painkillers. But they often improve if the patient is treated with an antidepressant.

Drugs such as ibuprofen and paracetamol are said to be less effective for women, not because they work differently in men but because they have no effect on the psychological aspect of pain.

But men don't have it all their own way. A woman is three times more likely to have her recurring headache correctly diagnosed as migraine and treated appropriately. Perhaps this is because migraine is best diagnosed by a careful analysis of the patient's description of their symptoms, and women are better at delivering that analysis. A chimpanzee with a clipboard could get the classic history of a one-sided thumping pain, triggered by stress, tiredness or caffeine, accompanied by nausea and preceded by a bit of visual blurring, from a woman. All it would get from a bloke with the same headache would be, 'I'll tell you one thing, Cheetah, it bloody hurts.'

Things might improve after some aspirin and a nap in a quiet dark room. For the chimp at least.

WHAT IS IT WITH PARAMEDICS AND 'INFORMED CONSENT'?

THEY SAY PEOPLE are funny, but I prefer the term 'mad'. I had cause to reflect on this earlier in the week as I was confronted in our waiting room by a father carrying the limp form of his young child.

Imagine *you* have a six-year-old daughter, and you treat her to a KFC takeaway. Let's further imagine that while gorging herself on a family-sized bucket, your daughter gets a chicken bone stuck in her throat and starts choking.

Now, what would *you* do?

Do the numbers '999' figure anywhere?

Well, when that all happened to little Sophie Wackles, dad didn't do the obvious. Instead, he carried her a quarter mile down the road to Bleak House and stood there in the doorway like the Creature from the Black Lagoon holding the lifeless remains of another victim.

Luckily, it didn't take *us* long to realise that the drooling and rapidly deteriorating kiddie needed to be shifted to a brightly-lit room staffed by girls and boys who had paediatric laryngoscopes and weren't afraid to use them.

So we rang 999 for those who are clad in green and first on the scene. I refer, of course, to our esteemed friends and colleagues the paramedics.

To be fair to them, they were with us inside five minutes. A good start – no time to lose, you'd have thought. A&E here we come, blues and twos, the whole thing.

Not so. The next thing I heard wasn't the squeal of gurney wheels on a laminated floor and the flap flap flap of the waiting room door as it caught the breeze of the departing stretcher. It was, 'Hello, Sophie. My name's Zoolander. How are you feeling? Is it OK if we move you from the examination couch onto this nice blue trolley?'

WTF? Guys, she's *six*. And even if she *was* in a position to give informed consent she isn't actually able to talk BECAUSE THERE'S A FUCKING CHICKEN WING WEDGED BETWEEN HER VOCAL CORDS! However, her mother *is* running around my waiting room like the proverbial and entirely non-ironic headless chicken, screaming, 'Help! Help! Help! Won't somebody save my baby!' Could you possibly consider that as implied parental consent and get her the hell out of here and into your big yellow taxi?

And this is absolutely not the time to start filling in your time sheets. Not while she's going a bit blue around the gills. I don't usually worry about much but even my 'Give a Toss-o-Meter' was starting to register high levels of giving a toss. Just get up and go. Really. Go to Casualty. Go directly to Casualty. Do not pass 'GO'. Do not collect 200 brownie points for asking a moribund child meaningless questions.

Eventually they left.

The end of this morning's surgery brought another similar run-in.

Mrs Peggotty buzzed through with a call from the 999 service. They had their hands on a middle-aged patient of ours who had started acting oddly at work – rambling slightly, unsteady on his feet and unable to focus on his computer screen. His BP was a sky-high 240/120 and – insofar as he was coherent at all – he was refusing to go to hospital, even though:

(i) He is a known hypertensive

(ii) He is a heavy smoker

(iii) He'd had his first stroke at the age of 43

(iv) He was having problems focusing on his PC screen.

'We're going to drop him off at home and you can visit him there,' said the voice on the end of the phone.

'Like fu.... er, like hell you are,' I said. 'Bring him to the surgery, I'll see him immediately.'

There was a pause. 'Hang on, doc,' said the voice. 'We'll just ask if that's OK with him.'

Ten minutes later the ambulance pulled up outside Bleak House. There's no way our hypertensive, CVA-surviving smoker could have given reasoned consent to anything, including the question of whether he wanted to be dropped at home, hospital or here. He was walking and talking alright, but he was walking sideways and talking gibberish, despite being stone-cold sober. I checked his BP. It was now 230/110. I had a quick peek into his eyes with the ophthalmoscope: no signs of papilloedema or retinopathy. So far so good. But he still needed to be taken to hospital.

'This is a no brainer,' I said. 'This patient should be in hospital now having his BP lowered while he's under obs.'

'Obs' are what the soap operas call 'observation' and what we call 'having a student nurse reading *Heat* magazine somewhere at the other end of the ward.'

'He doesn't want to go to hospital,' said one of the paramedics.

'He doesn't know what day of the week it is, never mind what's best for him,' I said. 'I'm telling you to take him to hospital. Tomorrow he'll wake up and thank you.'

If they'd taken him there in the first place, despite his protestations, he'd have walked straight in, just like he did to my surgery – but that would have conflicted with his right to choose; in this case, to take his chances at home.

I'm all for patient choice but I don't expect patients to be asked to risk their lives for it.

PAPILLOEDEMA, RETINOPATHY, CVA AND CONSENT

IT MIGHT HELP to explain a few terms from the above piece. Papilloedema is swelling of the optic disc inside the eye. Retinopathy is non-inflammatory damage to the retina. Both can be caused by uncontrolled high blood pressure, which can lead to a stroke or even death if left untreated. A stroke (or CVA – cerebrovascular accident) is a rapid loss of brain function due to a failure of blood supply to part of the brain because a blood vessel has either been blocked by a torn-off piece of its lining or has split along its length as a result of the pressure it's been subjected to over the years, causing a leak or haemorrhage. Hypertension contributes to both, but especially the latter. When a patient's BP suddenly goes through the roof, bad things can happen very quickly.

There's no such thing as 'normal' blood pressure as it naturally varies depending on circumstances. A typical resting BP for a healthy person would be in the order of 120/80; the '120' and '80' here refer to the height of a column of mercury that would be supported by the pulse, measured in millimetres and as seen in old fashioned blood pressure machines. The first number indicates the pressure produced by each individual heartbeat and the second the resting pressure in the system between them.

As blood pressure is so variable, no-one should be diagnosed as having high blood pressure – in other words, 'hypertensive' – unless their BP has been measured on three or four occasions (preferably by the same doctor or nurse using the same machine) over a period of weeks; dangerously high blood pressure is extremely rare.

Most cases have no underlying cause and we give them the slightly odd title of 'essential hypertensives' as, essentially, there's nothing else wrong with them. A few cases, around 5% of the total, are the result of kidney problems, hormone imbalances and structural abnormalities of the blood vessels themselves.

There are links between essential hypertension and family history, obesity, drug use, excessive salt intake and smoking. You can't choose your parents but you can address all the other issues if need be.

For a definition of 'Informed consent', à la Sophie Wackles, you could try visiting www.NHS.uk, where a search for those terms will reveal 258 articles in the NHS Choices section alone. But basically it means that you are provided with all the necessary information about a given medical procedure and then asked if you're happy for us to do it to you. Parents can usually give consent to treatment on their child's behalf. If you can't give informed consent (because, say, you're in the throes of a stroke – are you listening, paramedics?), then things get more complicated, but the general idea is that you should act in the patient's best interests, even if that sometimes means ignoring cries of 'leave me alone'.

IS IT ALWAYS MEA CULPA?

'IT'S LIKE Latin lessons all over again,' I said, looking up from my paper. 'And I was never any bloody good at that, either.'

Sami Patel was over in the other corner of common room, devouring *Top Gear* magazine with the slavering concentration of a teenaged boy perusing a copy of *Penthouse*.

He looked up. 'Do you think I should get one of these?' He waved the magazine at me – it had a preposterous yellow sports car on the cover. I ignored him and pressed on.

'This Heart UK stuff about cholesterol, it's bloody ridiculous,' I said. 'It says here that doctors are failing to deal with a rising tide of ill-health caused by cholesterol-related disease. It's like my old Latin school reports... could do better.'

Sami looked up. '*We're* failing?' he said. 'I don't think so.'

'Me neither,' I said. 'I spend half my life cajoling patients about their lifestyle, and half my budget on cholesterol-busting drugs. I chase all their sodding cardiovascular targets...'

'For the QOF points,' said Sami.

'For the QOF points, yes,' I said. 'How else am I going to put the bread and low-cholesterol spread on my table? And I refer anyone with the slightest chest twinge to a cardiologist. How the *hell* can *I* be failing?'

'The punters have wised up, too,' agreed Sami. 'They know that a heart attack needs an ambulance. A few of them even take the drugs I prescribe, rather than flushing them down the loo like they used to.'

'I can't see how things are worse,' I said. 'When was the last time you encountered the coronary end-game? You know, a night call for a blue and breathless patient with cardiac failure, lungs filling with fluid?'

'Well, we don't do nights any more,' said Sami.

'No, but you get the drift. This is just headline-grabbing bollocks. Cardiac care has been *transformed* in recent years. Look, they even admit that mortality from coronary heart disease is falling. OK, our rates are still up there with the worst in Western Europe, but there's more to this than cholesterol. We don't eat like the French and we smoke more than most.'

I read on. '*Thirty thousand more deaths could be prevented annually in the UK by increasing treatment*, they say. Well, sure, but there's only so much money to spend and so many pills patients can pop. *The number of people living with heart disease is increasing…* Ah! I get it. We're preventing the deaths, so the survivors have to live with their dodgy tickers.'

'Well, if we can't completely prevent illness, it's surely only fair that we should ensure a swift *coup de grâce* instead,' said Sami. 'The government are never going to be happy until everyone lives to 120 and works to 110, so we can all pay the taxes they need to keep themselves in limos and duck islands.'

'*Tackling cholesterol is key to the nation's heart health*, says the chairman of Heart UK,' I said. 'The government must stop dragging its heels or we will live to regret it, apparently.'

'Or not, obviously,' said Patel.

He rolled up his *Top Gear* and left, girding his loins for an afternoon of incontinent old ladies and vomity kids. I just sat there, thinking. Cholesterol levels have taken over from bowel movements as the nation's health obsession. My patients don't need their awareness raised, they need their anxieties allayed.

FEW THINGS MORE ALARMING

'HANG ABOUT THERE, DOC,' said Mr Winkle, during our consultation this morning. 'Only I just need to whip out my…'

I recoiled instinctively, my head swimming with visions of him presenting me with his poxed organ and a worried expression.

But no. In fact, he whipped out the only thing which approaches a poxed organ in terms of its ability to alarm a GP – and I include in that a sheaf of internet printouts or a never-ending list of symptoms. It was his Dictaphone.

'Let me just…' he said, putting on his reading glasses and studying the device with great concentration. 'I think you press it here… no. Is that it? Er… can you have quick look at it for me, doc?'

He handed it over – a sleek little digital thing made by Sony with buttons the size of pinheads.

'Have you tried pressing here where it says "Record"?' I said. 'I'm no technical whiz myself, but it seems fairly straightforward.'

'D'you know, I can't bleeding see it!' he said. 'Bleeding opticians, eh? Can you…? D'you mind if I…?'

It's not often that patients ask to record us, but if they do you can rest assured that they have our full attention: when you attend brandishing recording equipment, you might as well have 'potential litigant' tattooed on your forehead.

It's getting more common, apparently, but in the case of Mr Winkle – and indeed in most cases, I believe – it's nothing to do with attempted medico-legal intimidation but more to provide the patient with an *aide mémoire*.

Which is hardly surprising: research indicates that the average patient's recollection of our words of wisdom is abysmal. Apparently, you only ever remember three things per consultation: something from the beginning, something from the middle and something from the end. So that's: 'Hello', 'It's a virus' and 'Goodbye'. No wonder the phrase, 'I saw the doctor today' is so often juxtaposed with, 'and what a bloody waste of time it was, too!'

Presumably, we should shoulder at least some of the blame for failing to make each consultation adequately memorable – but then, it's not easy to turn five minutes of ingrowing toenail into a tale to dine out on for years.

One of many training hoops the would-be GP has to jump through these days includes videotaped consultations with patients. To float the trainer's boat, the tape should show the registrar attempting to check the patient's recall and understanding of the interaction. It can be amusing: I saw one trainee end his appointment by earnestly asking the patient: 'Can you remember what I've just said to you?'

He received the reply: 'Jeez, doc, your memory's worse than mine.'

Of course, this 'confirm, recall and understanding' box, like so many others, is really ticked only for exam purposes.

In real life, a grunted, 'OK?' or a quizzically-raised eyebrow is the best you'll get.

I have tried the approved method once. Having elegantly teased out a patient's symptoms and discussed, at length, and in a clear and sympathetic way, how his psyche (stressed and in turmoil) was affecting his stomach (twingeing and diarrhoeal), I decided to confirm his grasp of the situation by getting him to explain it back to me.

'Certainly, doctor,' he said. 'You're saying I'm making it all up.'

Perhaps this offers some insight into the real reason why patients suffer consultation amnesia. Maybe clichéd phrases from the GP induce in them a reflex spasm which inhibits the memory. So perhaps we shouldn't knock the Dictaphone approach; after all, while the patient may switch off, the tape will keep running and when he plays it back in the comfort of his home possibly he'll realise that although the doctor did spout platitudes, at least they were accurate platitudes, because he did feel better in the morning and aspirin did help.

If not, and he ends up in hospital, then... sorry. Hopefully, his amnesia will extend to him forgetting the number of his solicitor.

WHY DO PATIENTS ATTACK THEIR GPS?

GAVIN THE LOCUM was back in this week, as the Senior Partner has gone on his annual two-week pilgrimage to Gstaad. Apparently, this year the snow is lovely, the royals are in town and he's hoping to enjoy a slopeside *glühwein* or two with Charles. Well, it certainly beats my Tesco 'dark roast' instant coffee with Sami Patel.

The week before, Gavin had been working at a practice in a town not far away, standing in for a GP who had been attacked by a patient. The patient had visited the doctor and demanded to be signed off sick on specific dates in the future. Given that illness doesn't really work like that, the doc had quite rightly refused. At which point, the patient threw a bag of shopping at the GP and punched him in the face.

Remember that £97 million government scheme announced a few years back aimed at 'protecting frontline NHS staff from violence'?

No, me neither. I wonder if it has occurred to the government that one reason we need this protection is because of the extended hours imposed on us by, er, the government? Those extra hours are likely to be worked in isolation, at night, and in health centres that might as well have a flashing neon sign above them saying, 'Class A Drugs – All-U-Can-Steal'.

Apparently, healthcare workers are now being supplied with personal attack alarms. I'm not sure if they've been issued yet, but I certainly haven't had one. That's despite a BMA survey of 3,000 doctors from 2007 in which a third of GPs said they had been assaulted at work.

Thankfully, the physical abuse I receive from patients tends to be pretty tame. Some of it's even funny, in a way – like the time, not long ago, that an elderly and intractably constipated chap chucked a packet of medication at me whilst shouting, '…and you can shove these up your arse!'

Which was true, because they were suppositories.

The only other recent excitement in our practice involved the Senior Partner sending out an e-alert requesting immediate assistance. Instantly, doctors, nurses and receptionists converged on his room, expecting him to be grappling with an axe-wielding maniac. To our disappointment, he was quietly consulting a well-known, frequently attending, time-consuming heartsink who, though a source of mental anguish, never threatens us any physical harm. The SP's elbow had inadvertently leant on the alarm button (yes, we have alarm buttons in our surgeries), which is what can happen when you doze off during a consultation.

Verbal abuse, on the other hand, is pretty common, and ranges from frank insults to subtle slights. Among the best of the latter came from the patient who I indulged with 20 minutes of prime consulting time. I played it by the book, just like a proper Royal College GP – probably because we were on video as part of the practice's training reaccreditation, and the standard 30 seconds of perfunctory chat about his itchy bottom, the quick prescription and the gentle shove out of the door doesn't give the inspecting team much to get their teeth into.

So I patiently explored his ideas, established his concerns, discussed his expectations and 'involved him in the treatment strategy', as per the utterly ridiculous guidelines. And only after all of that guff did I stand up to shove him out of the door.

At which point he uttered those crushing words that deflate every GP: 'Thanks anyway, doctor.'

'Thanks', fine. But 'anyway'? The subtle barb hung in the air like a bad smell for a long time after he had left – a reminder that there was something rotten about that consultation.

It only cleared as I immersed myself in the final patient of the day, Mr MacStinger.

'I've come to you, Dr Copperfield,' he said, 'because the last doctor I consulted was bloody useless. Now, I'm going to need some antibiotics, a scan and a referral to see a top specialist...'

I was nodding along, as though I was giving all of this serious consideration, when I noticed that the previous consultation had, in fact, been with me. True, it was some time ago, and 'Dr Bloody Useless' has had his hair cut and perhaps put on some weight since then. But his diagnosis and attitude remained the same.

So I'd just been insulted, and was quite possibly hurt. What about an apology? Ah. Any hope of that evaporated as I noted, for the first time, that the patient was considerably bigger than me, was heavily tattooed, had no neck and appeared to be a bit cross.

Now, where's that personal attack alarm?

SATURDAY'S KIDS

EVERY COUPLE OF months I do a Saturday morning shift at our branch surgery on the outskirts of town.

It's a squat, pebble-dashed affair which nestles between some nice new two-bedroom flats with IKEA kitchens and the Staffordshire Cross council estate it was originally built to serve.

The idea is that our Saturday surgery offers GP access to the young, fit, childless, affluent, floating voter commuters who live on the posh side of the line into the nearest city and find it 'difficult' to get to see a doctor during working hours.

In truth, it's just a politically-motivated scam. Anyone from the estate without an appointment gets turned away – even the ones who might actually be ill. Their complex psychosocial problems and tendency to somatise are deemed unworthy of a Saturday morning consultation. They must ring the out-of-hours service on their stolen iPhones and grovel for their antibiotics, opiates and sleeping pills. The PCT is adamant that these sessions are reserved for patients who might find it inconvenient to attend during the week – nice, middle-class people who make appointments and have jobs to go to, like the people who work for the PCT.

This is bad enough, but my real problem with it is the fact that the PCT has insisted that there be a proper doctor on the premises throughout the session, which starts at 8am and grinds on until 1pm. 'Proper' doctor is defined as 'GP partner' – medics further down the food chain don't count.

So while the registrars, locums, assistants, nurses and receptionists come and go, Muggins here has to sit through the whole shooting match.

Plan A was some five-minute appointments at 8am and a few more at midday, giving me time to slip off for a leisurely decaf latte and skinny muffin in the interim. Unfortunately, this was scuppered a while back by practiceführer Jane Carstone. She took over my bookings and, to ensure my uninterrupted attendance, now timetables 18 appointments for me at 15-minute intervals.

Some doctors are all in favour of the quarter-hour slot. The thinking is, you can address the patient's unspoken agenda, you can delve into the depths of their psyche while adopting a concerned and supportive expression. Then, and only then, do you feel comfortable in handing out a prescription for salicylic acid gel to treat their verruca.

But as far as I'm concerned you can hold a patient upside down and shake them for seven or eight minutes at the most before you've got all the QOF money out of their pockets that you're going to get. Anything beyond that is purely onanistic.

Once I've done the smoking nag, the smear nag, the chlamydia nag and the flu jab nag, coded them as 'not depressed', entered a BP reading of 148/88 or less, recorded their ethnic background and put all the chubby ones on Orlistat, I'm bored as shitless as they're going to be after their third or fourth dose. (A side effect of Orlistat is sudden bowel movement.)

So I need a Plan B. The best I can come up with at the moment is to rebrand our filing clerk Stella as a 'consultant wellness adviser'. 'Consultant' trumps 'GP' any day, but especially at weekends. She can hold the fort after midday – I've got a pub to go to.

NITS FOR CASH

'DOCTOR OFFERS CASH for head lice,' said Gavin, our locum, almost to himself. 'Wish I had head lice.'

The kettle clicked, he made a cuppa and walked back out to surgery, shaking his head. Contrary to popular belief, GPs are not all swimming in cash; Gavin drives an eight-year-old Golf, owns precisely one jacket and – thanks to his predilection for spawning vast numbers of progeny with women who then leave him – is always boracic lint.

I picked up his *Times* from the draining board. To my surprise, it was true: apparently, a doctor at Bristol University wanted 300 lice for research into a new shampoo and was offering a bounty of £1 per nit.

Presumably, there was a serious scalp-parasite shortage in the West Country.

For a moment, I imagined the sort of excitement this story might generate in the likes of Kyle Chuzzlewit and his graffiti *antagonistes*, if any of them read *The Times*. Hereabouts, lousy children are common, the parasitic stronghold being loosened only by a counter-epidemic of No1 skinhead haircuts, typically including a Union Jack pattern shaved into the back of the scalp. (The boys have their hair styled quite short, too.) But if nits means prizes, I can see the average household figuring out that Wayne and Chantelle's itchy scalps might keep the family in pizza for, well, a week or so.

These ideas are like buses, actually. A while back, Dr Andrew Wakefield – he of MMR infamy – was supposedly offering kids £5 for giving a blood sample.

In my average surgery, they're lucky if they get a two-minute play with some pathogen-riddled toys while I extract the details of today's panic from mum before a cursory examination, an ear-boxing for troubling me with a cold and on to the next child. True, the occasional plucky little soldier who says 'Aaaaah' without puking over my shirt gets an 'I was brave at the doctor's' sticker, and those who let the nurse jab them without swearing are rewarded with a sweetie. But a *fiver* for a few drops of blood? If my local horrors got wind of that, everyone in the entire town would look like extras from *Twilight*.

The idea of paying patients isn't as radical as you might think. Financial inducements have for some time been suggested as a way of improving 'compliance' in patients with mental health or drug problems. As we know, some health evangelists have even gone as far as suggesting that patients should be offered cash incentives to attend routine health checks – and, as *I've* said, if this sounds like the most stupid idea ever in the history of medicine that's because it is. You don't need to be a behavioural psychologist to realise that the kind of punter who will be lured by financial rewards is also the sort who will spend it on a double lard burger within three minutes of leaving the surgery, or that the chances of him taking all the blood-pressure and cholesterol-busting treatments that he will inevitably need are the same as the chances of him attending follow-up appointments when the bungs run out: zero.

I'm not denying that bribery has a place in modern medicine, though. Indeed, I've been known to hand over cash to a patient purely to short-circuit a potentially lengthy and difficult consultation.

Only last week, Mrs Murdstone was in with her usual catalogue of symptoms, complaints and maladies.

'I've brought my list,' she announced, as people seem to do whenever we GPs are running an hour late and suffering an intractable tension headache.

As I've mentioned before, Rule One in such skirmishes is to gain control of said list, even if this involves some metaphorical, or even actual, arm-twisting. Leaning forward, I noticed that item 8, subsection C, was the reminder: 'Get doctor to sponsor my parachute jump'.

'Can I just see that?' I said, reaching over and grabbing the sheet. 'Let's see… right… you haven't got TB, I think it's just a slight cough… hmmm, I doubt that getting pins and needles in the mornings means you're getting multiple sclerosis, it's probably just, you know, pins and needles… er, have you been abroad recently? No, so I think we can rule out yellow fever… da da da da da… typhoid… rheumatism… No, I think you're in the clear. Oh! I see you're doing a jump for charity? How does a tenner sound? Good. And if I hand it over now, do you think we could leave it there? Excellent, here we are.'

It was the best £10 I've ever spent.

Come to think of it, I'd be happy to stump up the cash in other situations: for instance, if patients would agree to be bribed into never asking for allergy tests for symptoms that have everything to do with anxiety and nothing to do with allergy; or never opening a tissue to reveal something luminous and sticky they hawked up two days ago; or never coughing so exaggeratedly that they make themselves retch in the hope that this might act as the tipping point in my deliberations over whether to prescribe an antibiotic; or never using the words 'dizzy', 'tired' or 'magazine article' in my consultations; or doing any one of a hundred other things that make me wonder why I do this job, a thought that passes only when I remember that:

> a) I once wanted to save lives
> and
> b) I now want to earn enough money to bribe patients to stop doing the things that make me wonder why I do this job.

Here's a genuinely revolutionary idea, though. In recent years, government policy has, at times, devolved NHS budgets to those most attuned to patients' needs i.e. we family doctors. These days, we're amateur accountants – hence ideas like GP fund-holding and practice-based commissioning. Transpose 'patient wants' for 'patient needs' and you might as well give the dosh directly to the punter.

It's genius. Divvy up the NHS budget to give Mr and Mrs Average £X,000 a year to finance *all* their health problems. They can blow it all on facelifts or save it for a peaky day – the choice is theirs. And when the coffers are empty and they can't afford this clot-buster or that cancer wonder drug, they've only got their own bad book-keeping and/or bad luck to blame. NICE, the government and, most importantly, GPs are off the financial hook.

IN CASE OF EMERGENCY — JUST WAIT AND SEE

MRS PEGGOTTY WAS sticking up another one of her posters in the entrance vestibule when I arrived for work this morning.

It showed a grey-skinned and rather miserable-looking chap with what looked like a belt pulled tight around his chest.

'A CHEST PAIN IS YOUR BODY SAYING CALL 999,' said a slogan next to him. For added emphasis, a second slogan added: 'DOUBT KILLS. CALL 999 IMMEDIATELY.'

'Must we fill the place with this stuff, Mrs Peggotty?' I said. 'I mean, must we?'

'Yes, we most certainly must, Dr Copperfield,' she said. 'Doubt Kills. It says so here. And we wouldn't want that, now, would we?'

'Well, the fact is…' I said.

But she was gone in a haze of Elizabeth Taylor White Diamonds.

Mrs Peggotty's poster was supplied by the British Heart Foundation. The charity was moved to produce them after carrying out a survey which found that 42 per cent of people with chest pain will 'wait and see' if it gets better. Given that one third of people having heart attacks die before reaching hospital, you can see the rationale behind 'Doubt Kills'. But 'chest pain' covers an enormous multitude of sins, and it is *not* necessarily YOUR BODY SAYING CALL 999.

And – actually – we really *don't* want everyone who suffers from any chest pain, regardless of context, to ring for an ambulance; if everyone took that advice seriously, they'd have to wait a week for a paramedic and if they survived *that* it wouldn't make any difference because the hospitals would all be full anyway.

Sure, we'd maybe save the lives of a few people who wouldn't have otherwise bothered to call. But we'd lose lots of others who were patiently waiting in pieces by the sides of roads after car accidents.

The truth is, there's a world of difference between a 19-year-old non-smoker having sore ribs after he's coughed, and a fag-toting, diabetic pensioner with furred arteries suffering crushing central chest pain with associated sweating, vomiting and breathlessness.

Unfortunately, Sod's Law is that the first patient lives on Planet A (for Anxiety), and so responds to any twinge and media scare story by reaching for the phone over what is obviously non-cardiac pain, and the second lives on Planet B (for Bone-headedness) and ignores a genuine emergency.

There is, at least, some good news. Of those people who *do* decide to ring someone when they experience this sort of pain, the vast majority dial 999 – the percentage who'd call a reflexologist is a big, fat zero. This shows that, when the chips are down, you'll go for powerful clot-busting drugs over a foot massage every time.

That said, if you do go down the 999 route and end up in hospital, your Pavlovian desire to be near defib paddles the moment your chest twinges has other disadvantages: hospital doctors tend to assume the worst. So, despite your ECG and blood tests being normal, if you used the words 'chest' and 'pain', you may well be treated as a cardiac patient until proved otherwise. In the interim, while awaiting tests, you're downgraded from 'heart attack' to 'angina' and force-fed a cocktail of heart drugs 'just in case'.

This is all fine and dandy, except for the fact that when the cardiologist eventually gives you the all-clear he inevitably forgets to give you permission to stop popping the pills. It's only about five years later that the penny drops, when I summon you to the surgery to clarify why your medical summary states 'All cardiac investigations normal', whereas your prescription record suggests the opposite. Unfortunately, by now your coronaries *have* actually furred up, so the day after I tear up your prescription, you drop dead.

It's a bugger, this job.

And not least because the real issue in general practice is the opposite to the one identified by the British Heart Foundation. For every patient who delays seeking medical help for a potentially serious symptom, there are hordes who attend urgently at the first sign of… well, anything.

So my emergency surgery is full of patients who have vomited once, or sprouted a single blotch that afternoon, or developed a headache half an hour ago. In which case, it's probably a virus, a virus and a virus, respectively. Yes, it *might* be meningitis or a brain tumour, but you just can't tell that early in an illness's evolution.

So, sometimes, that 'wait and see' policy derided by the British Heart Foundation wouldn't go amiss. Which is why I was delighted to note that there was one survey respondent who, despite severe chest pain, 'Wouldn't call 999 under any circumstances'. This shows that stoicism isn't completely dead. Even if the patient is.

SMOKING

LIKE MOST GPS, I live some distance from where I work.

There are many reasons for this, but mostly it's because I don't really want to be consulted about your suppurating ulcer while Mrs C and I are trying to enjoy a lasagne and insalata verde supper at Luigi's Trattoria.

Unfortunately, there's no decent supermarket where I live, so every fortnight or so I find myself browsing through the aisles in the mega Tesco down the road from the surgery.

Which is where I was when Mrs Skewton chanced upon me last night.

'Ooh, hello, doctor!' she said, leaning over to stare into my trolley. 'Fancy seeing you… ooh, tut, tut, who's a naughty boy, then? A pint of double cream? A giant-size pork pie? A family pack of Mars Bars? I'd have thought you were more of a brown rice and reduced-fat raisins sort of a chap!'

'Yes, well, I really must…'

'Because didn't you say to my Dave just the other week that he needed to cut down on the curry and lager?'

Your Dave would regard the entire contents of my trolley as a light snack, I thought. 'Well, the Mars Bars… ah… well, obviously, they're not for me. They're for… er… the kids… not my kids of course, they're for… er… other kids… er… we're going to a party…'

'And look at this, doctor! Chocolate fudge brownies! Four bottles of wine!'

'Erm… we're having friends round to dinner and…'

'Ben and Jerry's… what is it? Ben and Jerry's Caramel Chew-Chew? *Doctor*!'

At which point, I took the only option open to me, and said loudly, 'Anyway, did those suppositories sort out your Nobbys?'

Mrs Skewton abruptly developed a keen interest in the opposite shelf and I made my getaway.

At least she didn't catch me smoking. I don't actually smoke, but apparently more than two thousand doctors do, despite the well-known health risks associated with the habit.

Shocking though this figure is, I suspect it's an underestimate; apart from its familiar health effects, smoking also causes shrivelling of that part of the brain involved in telling the truth.

It's probably even worse among nurses. After all, they get more coffee breaks than doctors, and being hooked on caffeine is a match-strike away from being a nicotine addict. Besides, when you spend much of your day emptying bedpans, using fags to destroy your sense of smell must seem like a good idea.

Which prompts the question: should GPs really feel so guilty about their lifestyle choices? I think not. Many of the problems that traditionally bedevil the medical profession are the result of doctors stupidly playing up to the role of model citizens. The more virtuous we pretend to be, the harder we fall, which is why the public seems particularly unforgiving when we demonstrate human weakness, such as when we make mistakes, want to reduce working hours or groan when you whip out a list.

Far better for all concerned that we doctors admit to being mere mortals. And I don't see anything paradoxical or unprofessional in a lardy GP asking patients to lose weight, a slobbish doc advising exercise, or a ciggie-toting professor of respiratory medicine warning about smoking. After all, the 'Do as I say, not as I do' approach has served most parents and their offspring perfectly well over the years.

So I shall continue to indulge in the odd scoop of ice cream, add sugar to my coffee and let my gym membership lapse. Because, although my conscience isn't entirely clear, my attitude is. Patients are more likely to trust a flawed, real-life GP than a sanctimonious automaton. So let me eat cake. You can put that fag out, though.

WHY GPS SOMETIMES GET IT SO WRONG

I THOUGHT DR EMMA looked unusually flustered when I passed her in the corridor this morning, but when I asked her if she was OK she shuddered and ducked into the ladies' loo.

As usual, Sami Patel was in the know.

'She's just been told that a woman she diagnosed with the menopause has given birth to a bouncing baby boy,' he said with a grin. 'Could happen to anyone, I suppose.'

It reminded me of another story I read recently, about a young boy whose nine years of deafness was not, as his doctors had suggested, caused by wax. This became apparent when the tip of a long-forgotten cotton bud was removed from his ear, completely curing his problem.

So, two people with unexpected items popping out of bodily orifices, both of which prompt the same question: why are we GPs so dumb? How can we get things *so* wrong?

Believe me, it's easy.

Take those two examples.

The offending cotton bud would have been fossilised in a nine-year sediment of wax, cruelly misleading the GP, and the menopausal child-bearer's symptoms – tiredness, bloating, absent periods, weight gain, emotional wobbliness – are the same as those for pregnancy. As Sami said, it could happen to anyone.

The surprise is not that there are so many 'Dumb-ass GP' headlines but that there are so few.

Consider the sheer volume of cases we deal with. I see about 40 patients every day, many presenting multiple problems and some smuggling in relatives beneath the receptionist's radar to bypass the appointment system. That's about 9,000 clinical dilemmas posed each year, against a distracting background of *en passant* gripes about the waiting room decor, about GPs no longer doing out-of-hours and toddlers puking on the carpet.

Then, as I've said, there's the fact that we see illness at its earliest stages, when it's most difficult to diagnose. So, 'I'm worried about my child, she's vomited twice in the last ten minutes,' poses a problem – and not just because I've got to clean my carpet again. It's more that the list of possible diagnoses encompasses just about every condition known to man.

'It's probably just a virus,' I'll say.

Unfortunately, mum inevitably forgets the 'probably' bit, and also the fact that I told her to ring me if the little girl gets any worse. Which is why, when the classical symptoms appear later and the white-coated hospital heroes cure her daughter's meningococcal septicaemia, the papers will deride me as a numbskull or an incompetent or a heartless bastard, or all of the above.

Let's suppose I *can* diagnose you quickly – maybe you are unlucky enough to have developed a DVT as a souvenir of a long-haul flight. You'll be prescribed the rat poison warfarin (that's no medical error, it's standard treatment). Warfarin requires regular blood tests and dose adjustments. Here's the routine: a nurse takes your blood, places it in the right tube and completes a form with the correct dosage details; the sample is safely transported to the lab where it is analysed by a machine, which churns out a precise blood thickness reading; this figure is correctly transcribed by a technician on to a report form, which is relayed back to the health centre; the GP reads it meticulously and correctly calculates the revised warfarin dose; the new instructions are carefully passed to the practice secretary, who then accurately conveys them to you. And you follow them to the letter.

A close analysis of this particular example reveals that an apparently straightforward process actually involves about 17 discrete steps. That's 17 potential sources of error – and, every day, *thousands* of GPs are involved in *scores* of these tasks. Number crunch these stats and you'll discover that there are billions of links each year in the medical chain.

Frankly, it's a miracle you're not all dropping like flies.

Despite this, the Department of Health recently announced it wanted to reduce serious medication errors by 40 per cent. (Why not 45%? Or 70%?)

Luckily GPs have access to the best error-spotters of all – patients, as in: 'Er, Dr Copperfield, you've accidentally septupled my immunosuppressant dose by prescribing it daily rather than weekly, but I forgive this potentially fatal error because you are overworked.'

Usually, it's not that serious, anyway – as in the case of Mr Fagin, who consulted me later that day.

'Basically, doctor,' he said, 'I'm feeling a bit stressed and I'd like some help.'

No problem. He clearly needed some relaxation exercises. I find a handout paints a thousand words – which was good news, because I was running late. I rifled through my leaflets, then thrust one in his hand with a cheery, 'See how you get on with that.'

Unfortunately, in my alphabetically-indexed leaflet file, R for *Relaxation Exercises* is right next to S for *Semen Analysis – How to Obtain Your Specimen*.

Which is the leaflet Mr Fagin received.

'I'm not being funny doctor,' he said, 'but how the hell is that going to help my stress levels?'

Rather well, I'd have thought.

NICKLEBY: THE FINAL CURTAIN

'I'VE STILL GOT that buzzing in my ear.'

Oh. Well, that's a bit disappointing.

'I think it's my somatisation disorder playing up.'

Some insight, then. Possibly.

'Because I've got my backache again, my headache…'

My mind wandered slightly. We've tried everything now, including engaging Mr Nickleby on a psychological level.

'…my dry skin, the belching, my itchy nipples…'

Underlying concerns, past traumas, or aberrant family dynamics might all be behind his constant worrying, but he won't hear a bar of it.

'…my tongue's a horrible colour, the catarrh's come back, my ankles are puffy…'

We've tried him on low doses of antidepressants, but he refuses to take, or refuses to tolerate, those.

'…the heartburn's awful, I'm getting palpitations and I've started bleeding from my back passage…'

Maybe we should give it another go, maybe the current psychological panacea of Cognitive Behavioural Therapy might make some headway… hang on. Rewind.

'What was that you just said?' I asked, suddenly alert, antennae twitching.

'About the palpitations?'

'No, no, the other thing?'

He thought for a second. 'Er, I've started bleeding from my back passage?'

Alarm bells. To his utter astonishment, I had him up on the couch in a flash for the rubber glove/KY jelly treatment.

Bugger me. There it was. A huge great mass in his rectum. Worse still, when I turned him round to examine his belly, I could feel a big, craggy liver.

Which meant the cancer had spread. The poor old sod.

'The somatisation disorder *is* playing up,' I said. 'But so is something else.'

That was the last I ever saw of him.

MISDIAGNOSING DEATH

I WAS CALLED out to Mrs Bangham's house the other morning. Her husband had been unable to wake her and, since she was 92, had feared the worst.

Given that she'd spent the last few months battling her terminal cancer, I took a death certificate with me.

When I got there, I found the old dear propped up in bed, eyes and mouth open, in a blue flannelette nightie. She was obviously dead, but just in case I went through the motions.

The first thing to do in these situations is to check for a pulse. If you are unable to find one, you spend 30 seconds listening to the chest for anything that might resemble a heartbeat. Half a minute is a long time and, believe me, in that situation *everything* – every creak from the central heating or floorboards – sounds like a heartbeat. Given that there was no pulse and no audible heart sounds, it was out with the torch (if we're trying to impress, we might use an ophthalmoscope). In a dead person, the pupils of the eyes will be wider than usual and won't react to a light shone directly into them.

Her pupils didn't change. Any patient who doesn't respond to a good shout or a prod, isn't breathing for themselves, has no detectable pulse and whose pupils are fixed and dilated is certainly dead.

(There are some rare conditions that can mimic death, but you've more chance of winning the lottery. Mind you, that happens to someone almost every week. Let me rephrase that...)

'I'm sorry, Mr Bangham,' I said. 'There's nothing I can do here.'

'At least she went in her sleep,' he said, wiping his eyes. 'It would have been our 70th wedding anniversary in March. But she had a good innings, the old girl.'

I wrote out a death certificate, called the undertakers and made Mr Bangham a cup of tea while we waited for them to arrive.

Then I left and, as I did so, I thought about my mate Steve from medical school who trained as a hospital doc and once famously pronounced an elderly man dead, only for the patient to open his eyes and demand a pint of Guinness. Even 20 years later, this is something Steve and I never, ever talk about. Well, *he* doesn't; I mention it from time to time.

As it happens, according to information recently obtained under the Freedom of Information Act by the BBC, an average of one person each year is pronounced dead but goes on to recover. And those figures cover only patients in hospital, where doctors have easy access to helpful gizmos such as heart monitors and brainwave recorders. There were no figures given for the lower-tech world of general practice, but common sense says it must happen once in a while. It's not something I've experienced yet, though I've had a few close calls. Many times in the past I've visited one of my 'terminals' and – on the basis that she had no blood pressure, pulse or indeed any measurable physiological parameter other than one death-rattle every few minutes – solemnly advised the family to start thumbing through the 'U' section of the *Yellow Pages*.

Next morning I arrive with suitably grave face to complete the formalities, only to find Nearly-Dead Nan swigging back a bottle of sherry and leading the family in a right old knees-up. I hurriedly shred the death certificate and say, sheepishly: 'She's obviously going to carry on for quite some weeks yet.'

Which also proves slightly inaccurate, as I discover when I get a call the next day to complete the cremation papers.

So I sympathise, a bit, with my mate Steve's embarrassment. It's bad enough when the rash I have confidently diagnosed as eczema turns out to be ringworm, or the badly-sprained wrist is actually a hairline fracture. Announcing that Mrs X has shuffled off this mortal coil and sending her off to be bagged and tagged, only for her to sit up in the morgue and demand a cup of tea, will do my credibility no good at all. Not to mention the real risk of suffering a lawsuit from a psychologically-scarred embalmer.

WHY ALL DOCTORS ARE TECHNOPHOBES

I SPENT MOST OF my lunch break trying to work out how to make a telephone call with the whizzy new mobile they sent me to replace the old one which the Senior Partner ran over with his Jaguar in the car park last week.

I don't know why they can't just make a phone which simply allows you to phone people you want to phone. I don't need 400 'apps' so I can run my central heating remotely, find out the current value of the Yen or discover what time it is in Bangalore, do I?

In the end I had to go in search of Henry Gowan, our posh young medical student, who understands this stuff.

I found him in the common room, entertaining what I felt were an inappropriately rapt Dr Emma and Registrar Lucie with tales of studently derring-do.

'Henry,' I said. 'Can I just borrow you a sec?'

He followed me to my room, and then followed my gaze to the shiny black mobile on my desk.

'Can you… work this for me please?' I said.

He picked it up. 'Nokia N96 with all the toys,' he said. 'That's actually a pretty cool phone. I mean, for an older guy.'

I wasn't sure which I objected to more – the note of surprise in his voice, or the description of me as 'an older guy'. Grudgingly, I swallowed my pride. 'Yes,' I said. 'But can you show me how to… you know, make a call?'

'Sure, Tone,' he said. 'I'll ring your direct line in here, yeah? I just need to…'

His thumb whizzed over the flat screen at a bewildering speed as he searched through the sodding thing's various menus and options.

'How's things, anyway?' I said, for something to say. 'Dr Patel keeping you busy?'

'Yeah, it's going great, thanks,' he drawled. 'Yeah, Sami's actually a great guy, you know? We're going up to town to, like, Ministry at the weekend.'

'What, the Ministry of Health?' I said. 'At the weekend? That sounds... keen.'

'No, like, *Ministry*, yeah? The Ministry of Sound? It's, like, a club? It's not actually that cool any more, but Sami wants to go, so...'

A vision of Sami Patel grooving on a dancefloor swam into my mind's eye. It was chased away by the ringing of the direct landline on my desk.

'There you go,' said Henry. 'Simples.'

Before he left, he kindly scribbled me an *aide mémoire* on my prescription pad in case I got bamboozled again.

I'm not alone in this technophobia. The fact is, most doctors can hardly refill their printer ink or set their Sky Plus – why people let us meddle with their vital organs I'm not really sure. It's not only mobile phones and remote controls that faze us, either – we're not exactly renowned for our keyboard skills. I dread meeting a patient with pseudopseudo-hyperparathyroidism or pneumonoultramicroscopic silicovolcanoconiosis, not because I'd miss the diagnosis but because it would take me the rest of the morning to type it into their medical record. My ponderous, two-fingered keyboard-bashing also reduces to somewhere near zero the chances of you and me exchanging e-mails about prescriptions for bendroflumethiazide or phenoxymethylpenicillin.

I'm not completely hopeless, mind. Unlike most NHS staff, I do actually have an NHS e-mail address. The last time I checked I had 7,000 unread messages, mostly offering d1sc0unt Vi@gr@ – perhaps because 'tony.copperfield@nhs.net' is the address I type into dodgy websites to divert junk mail away from my real account.

None of this stops various well-meaning types suggesting we adopt yet more complex systems. The medical 'think tank' the King's Fund hosts 'interactive multistakeholder events' and publishes lots of very boring documents like the recent page-turner, *Technology in the NHS*. It worries itself about the fact that, while most NHS surgeries have IT systems that patients can access to book an appointment online, only one surgery in ten actually uses them. Why? Because the last thing we need is punters surfing the web after midnight, deciding that they have an undiagnosed magnesium allergy, forwarding a copy of the website to us and blagging an urgent slot next morning. We'd rather see little old ladies who don't have wi-fi broadband but who *do* have genuine symptoms.

One King's Fund suggestion is that you use your camera phone to photograph your skin rash, send the pictures to us and wait for your prescription.

Whaaaat? A while back, our local prison spent serious money on a CCTV set-up, complete with studio lights, so they could sit scabby inmates in front of the camera and broadcast live to our skin clinic. The problem is that most of the time we *still* can't tell scabies from scurvy. A blurry late-night vidcap of your orange rash with the caption, 'Issit catchin?' is not going to help. Put it on YouTube if you like, just don't bother sending it to me.

I'm not a total luddite. I'd love to sign repeat prescriptions electronically, rather than watching my signature deteriorate into some sort of graffiti artist's tag after the first 50. I'd like to be able to send patients their test results or reminders about appointments by text message, too. And I'd really like patients to have some sort of smartcard for storing their main diagnoses and their current treatment.

Just kidding about that last bit, obviously. For one thing, it's happening – sort of – even as I type. And for another, I'm not in favour of it at all. The Summary Care Record is another of the government's Big Ideas. The plan is to have your medical records – and everyone else's – on a centralised database so that any medical professional can access it at any time. Which sounds sensible, as many of these ideas do, but isn't. It's a solution to a problem that doesn't exist. In a real emergency – which is when the information would be accessed – medical details aren't usually that hard to come by. We can ask you, for example, or your relatives, or your doctor. Besides, knowing you're allergic to Elastoplast isn't actually *that* important when, say, we're trying to defibrillate your heart. Factor in problems such as keeping the record up to date, anxieties about confidentiality and the enormous cost of the project and you pretty soon realise it's another dumb-ass, politically-driven white elephant. Someone who appears to need serious psychiatric help, known only as 'Department of Health spokesman' to avoid embarrassing his immediate family, said on the TV news that the NHS IT programme was 'saving time, lives and money'. Yeah, right. Buddy, I thought, as I watched him ramble on, you can phone me, fax me, text me, mail me, anything to make sure you get an urgent appointment. Meanwhile, I'm afraid this report is going to the only piece of GP technology I've mastered, the gadget that turns documents like this into soft fluffy bedding for the family hamster.

YOU *CAN* BE TOO CAREFUL

MRS STEERFORTH CONSULTED me this morning. She's a relatively new mum, and as she sat there in front of me, bouncing her two-year-old on her knee, I knew exactly what she was going to say.

'He was fine until half an hour ago,' she explained. 'Then he threw up. And he's been fine since.'

The boy gurgled happily, a picture of health.

'Uh-huh,' I murmured encouragingly, inviting her to offer the vital clue which had justified rushing a manifestly well child to the doctor's: the fact that he was also dropped on his head, perhaps, or had been caught red-handed with a bottle marked 'Nasty poison, keep away from Shiny Happy Toddlers'.

But none of this was forthcoming as I'd suspected it would not be, because none of it had happened. Instead, when the pause had become over-pregnant, she said, 'Well, you can't be too careful.'

So they say. Except that 'they' tend not to include GPs, who are on the receiving end of the Over-Cautious Culture. So we beg to differ: you can, indeed, be too careful.

This a colleague illustrated to me rather neatly, after I had recounted the two-year-old's consultation to him. We were involved in what NHS bureaucrats would describe as an Approved Postgraduate Educational Meeting comprising a Significant Event Audit – what the rest of us would describe as a pint down the pub.

'Oh yes,' he said, with authority, between slurps. 'You certainly can be too careful. I remember a chap with a boil who was worried he might have necrotising fasciitis. Insisted on rushing straight over to the surgery.'

'And?'

'He was killed by a car on the way there.'

I sent Mrs Steerforth on her way. With five minutes until my next patient, I decided to check my emails.

The top one was from Dr Emma.

Let me explain how fluffy our Emma is. Her 'doctors online' avatar is the Andrex puppy, she drinks decaf Diet Coke and wherever her chakras are, they're so finely balanced that she makes a meditating

Shaolin monk look like a candidate for an anger management class. When she invited a complementary 'therapist' along to give us a short and unintentionally hilarious talk about her work, I – being a creature of logic and reason – pointed out that I'd be more likely to eat one of the used nappies from that afternoon's Well Baby Clinic than allow her to lay hands on any patient of mine. Emma squirrelled the woman away for half an hour's 'post-traumatic' de-briefing and later forced me to send her a bunch of flowers to apologise for my outrageous behaviour.

So the following made my jaw drop somewhat, allowing delicious fragments of half-eaten Hob Nob (come *on* McVitie's) to spill onto the keyboard:

> 'Are anyone else's referrals to HealthPrime being bounced? One of my Chubby Mummies has just brought in a letter from them saying that they will only accept patients' second referral forms. So the patient has to book another appointment with me, to get an identical chit, before they get the help they need. I'll be taking this further.'

HealthPrime is the name for a scheme set up by the PCT to get the morbidly obese and patients who've recently had a heart attack to attend the local sports centre for some Personal Trainer input to help with weight loss and/or rehabilitation. Of course, the whole thing is a complete waste of time and money: the fat ones never see the programme through and, take it from me, patients who've survived their first heart attack need very little encouragement from anybody to change their lifestyle in an effort to prevent a second. If the Personal Trainer had a role there it would probably be to tell them to slow down and take things a little easier on the exercise bike.

That said, once we refer someone, that should be that. And the idea of Emma getting riled up enough to 'take things further' intrigued me, so I emailed back to make sure she hadn't got her Zang Fu meridians crossed. Was she sure that they hadn't meant to say they'd only accept referrals from Secondary Care – GP speak for the berks in white coats and bow ties? Her reply was virtually instant.

> 'No! It's as simple as it sounds. Patient comes to me, I refer them, they get knocked back and come back to see me again. I repeat exactly the same consultation I had ten days ago and send an exact copy of my original referral form – with a few rude comments added in the margin – to HealthPrime's office. This time, patient gets seen. I've had to do that three times in the last week.'

Emma? 'Rude' comments? No way. But then I read on:

> 'It's a fucking tarted-up fucking gym membership for fuck's sake.'

That outburst was, I assure you, as shocking as it gets. But it was unequivocal proof that my job can and does try the patience of a saint. Thrice over.

MR SWIDGER'S PRIVATE EXAMINATION

I STAYED AROUND AFTER work the other day to spend 30 minutes on a private examination of a Mr Swidger. By 'private' I mean he was paying for it as part of a job application process. He is hoping to become a mini-cab driver and medicals to do with work aren't 'General Practice', they're 'Occupational Health' so you don't get them free of charge.

He's not someone I'd ever travel with, at least not willingly. He has weapons-grade B.O., looks like Jabba the Hutt and is borderline simple. Still, you can't stop people from collecting fare-paying passengers just for being fat, smelly and dim-witted – the free market will see to that – so I got on with it.

At the end of a fabulous half-hour spent trying to hear his heartbeat though his barrel chest, recoiling at the smell wafting from the fungal rashes in every skin fold, wishing that I hadn't asked him to cough while I was checking for a hernia and wondering if they'd perfected a 'Snot and Sputum' Stain Devil designed to remove bodily fluids from linen pants, I finished with my usual question: 'Do you have any particular worries?'

'Only the price of this check-up,' he said. 'I mean, come on, eighteen quid for this? You doctors must be on a bloody fortune.'

'I'm sorry,' I said, 'but I think you must have misheard me. I didn't say *eighteen* pounds, I said *eighty* pounds. Maybe I should have tested your ears for wax a bit more carefully.'

I resisted the temptation to add that I'd spent a decade in training and even longer in practice and that this combination of knowledge and experience justified an hourly rate sufficient to cover my dry cleaning bills. Sure, eighty quid sounds pricey, but take that and divide it between four partners (private work done on surgery premises is practice income) and I end up with £20. Then that nice chap at 11 Downing Street will take 50% of the twenty, leaving me with £10 for half an hour's private work. Meanwhile, Mr Swidger has done nothing more than pass a driving test and will soon be earning more than that ferrying drunks from club to club in town in a clapped out Peugeot 405.

For a moment, he stared blankly at me. Then he silently wrote out a cheque for £80, shaking his head as he did so and handed it over with as much bonhomie as Hitler awarding Jesse Owens his gold medal.

Like many of my other patients, he is labouring under the belief that all GPs now earn well over a quarter of a million pounds a year. I wish. If the NHS afforded me a champagne lifestyle, why would I write this book?

SO HOW MUCH DO GPs EARN (AND HOW ARE THEY PAID)?

THE SHORT ANSWER is, on average, £106,000 a year before tax. So we're not pleading poverty. There are a few entrepreneurs who earn a lot more than this, and who get all the bad headlines, but they do have to work very hard for their wonga – they might run dispensing outfits (which means dispensing income), or take over and manage other practices, or do a lot of private work. This means long hours and a lot of responsibility, and I wouldn't fancy it, but it's their choice – unlike most NHS staff, who are employees, GPs are technically self-employed and can decide, within reason, how much work they want to do.

That said, our situation is a lot more complex than that of your average self-employed worker. (Years ago, one of the very first things I wrote for money was a guide to the payments system to which newly-qualified GPs could refer. It took me eight weeks to complete.)

After 1948, when the Minister of Health Aneurin Bevan opted to 'stuff GPs' mouths with gold' to get them to abandon their private practices and sign up to the newly introduced National Health Service, the monster that was the payment system grew and grew into a labyrinthine behemoth of bewildering complexity. The instruction manual known as the 'Red Book' ran to hundreds of pages.

GPs were paid a Basic Practice Allowance, just for setting up in practice, and then a sum of money per patient.

Some of their expenses – such as building costs, heating and lighting – were reimbursed, and bundled on top of that there was a complicated 'piece work' system where GPs got paid for performing some additional tasks known as 'Items of Service', like offering contraceptive advice and doing so-called 'minor' operations, which didn't form part of the 'traditional' GP provision.

They also received 'Seniority Payments' for getting older (or, some would say, surviving at least seven years in the job), 'Night Visit fees' for getting out of bed after 10pm (but not if all they did was answer the phone at four in the morning and give the standard, 'take two aspirins and call me again in the morning' advice – that was unpaid) and money for performing check-ups on elderly patients and new patients to their practices.

All of this changed in 2004 when a new contract was negotiated – although some GPs prefer to use the slightly more accurate term 'imposed'.

GPs are now contracted to offer 'General Medical Services' in exchange for a share of the total amount of money available to provide GP services across the NHS, a figure known as 'The Global Sum'.

The size of the share is determined by taking into account, among other things, the number and ages of the patients on the practice's list, the number of patients who join or leave the practice each year, the cost of hiring nurses and receptionists, and the number of 'deprived' patients in the area.

For most GPs, this contract left them better off than they had been before, with the intended average income rising from around £60,000 to nearer £90,000 per annum.

The minority who would be worse off were supported by a safety net known as M-PIG, the Minimum Practice Income Guarantee.

Are you with me so far? Good.

No sooner had the government agreed the Global Sum than it took a large chunk of it back again to fund the Quality & Outcome Framework (QOF) incentive scheme discussed earlier. As I said, there are a thousand QOF brownie points on offer, and because of a major miscalculation on the government's part almost every GP in the country gets almost all of them, just by doing all the stuff we previously did unpaid for years (often stuff we'd have to be on the edge of negligence to miss).

The General Medical Services thing and the QOF system are negotiated nationally. Larger practices can negotiate directly with their Primary Care Trust and enter into a contract to provide 'Personal Medical Services'. These contracts cover aspects of medical care that aren't included in the GMS contract but are still do-able by GPs and are needed in their area. For instance, one of my mates works in South East London and has about 2,000 Nigerians on his list, who all need travel vaccinations every time they go home, which is two or three times every year. So, travel vaccinations form part of his PMS contract.

The unintentionally generous QOF package – which saw GP earnings reach a peak in 2005 – resulted in an outcry, and the outcry resulted in pay cuts for GPs in 2006 (of 2.1%) and 2007 (of 1.5%). I'm not much of a betting man, but I don't expect to see another rise for quite some time.

OUT OF HOURS

THE OTHER KEY thing to talk about when discussing the New Contract and governmental cock-ups is out of hours (OOH) care.

When I was a boy (cue Dvorak's *New World*), GPs provided OOH care in emergencies.

By the time I began what I've laughingly come to call my 'career' in General Practice, the definition of an 'emergency' was showing real signs of slippage.

I started out young, keen and willing to visit patients anytime, day or night, but that feeling was soon knocked out of me by calls for, among other things, the morning-after pill at midnight. (The clue's in the name, girls.)

By 2004, politicians were promising that GPs would not only see genuinely ill people within 48 hours (neglecting to provide the space age technology by which it would be possible to ascertain before the fact who was and who was not 'genuinely ill'), but also people who merely 'believed themselves to be ill'. In my practice, this sometimes seems to equal the entire population. As a result, the government made it virtually impossible for patients who really needed to book regular appointments about long-term illnesses to get to see the same doctor each time – and it was clear that the concept of 'urgent' or 'emergency' care had vanished.

We were expected to provide instant access for even the most trivial conditions 24 hours a day, seven days a week – and, to a man and woman, we all hated it.

GPs were retiring early or leaving the NHS to work abroad, and far too few newly-qualified doctors wanted to replace them, opting instead for the greasy pole-climbing world of hospital medicine – which merely reinforces my point about how crappy a GP's working life had become.

Out of a clear blue sky, and to ease the passage of QOF, the government's crack team of world-class hagglers (I'm sorry, I am trying to keep a straight face, I really am) offered to allow GPs to 'opt out' of providing OOH care and make it the Primary Care Trust's problem.

Imagine the GPs' negotiators when faced with this offer. The thought process would have been along these lines:

> Blimey! They're going to let us off OOH! OK – must think straight, here. How much will the government want to take out of our wages in exchange for this massive, massive concession? Ten grand? Fifteen? Still, it'll be worth it. Sleep! And weekends off!

The government actually asked for £6,000 per GP. But don't worry, they said, we'll put a system in place that allows you to claim some OOH money in respect of the admin involved in opting out.

Back to the GP negotiation team:

> Y A A A A A H H H H H - B L O O D Y - HOOOOOOO!!!!!!!! A HUBBA-HUBBA-HUBBA!!! GET DOWN!!! GET RIGHT DOWN!!! YEAH!!! YEAH!!! YEEEEE-HAAAAH!!! THE GUYS BACK AT BMA HOUSE ARE NEVER, NEVER, *NEVER* GONNA BELIEVE THIS!

Actually, their response was probably more like, 'You drive a hard bargain, but in the interests of continuing dialogue, we're prepared to accept,' before excusing themselves, running to the nearest toilets and corpsing like a bunch of school kids who've just stuck a 'KICK MY SORRY ASS' note on the back of the Headmaster's jacket.

Meanwhile, entirely predictably, the national papers are now full of horror stories resulting from PCTs' attempts to provide OOH care for roughly £4 per patient, per year.

BURN OUT

I FOUND MYSELF in the Red Lion with the Senior Partner the other night. We'd escaped intact from a practice meeting and were slowly sinking a couple of pints and putting the world to rights, when he suddenly let out a heartfelt sigh.

'I dunno, Tony,' he said. 'I never thought I'd say this, but I'm starting to think about retirement. Charlie's away at uni now, so there's nothing keeping us here any more. D'you know, I've always fancied sailing round the world.'

'You haven't got a boat,' I said, 'and you don't know how to sail. Other than that, it's a great idea.'

'It's just, I've had enough of all the crap,' he said. 'When I began my career in general practice, I had an idea it could get pretty crappy. But I had no idea just how crappy. You'd have thought that, by now, with all my experience, I'd have reached some sort of crap plateau – but no, it continues to be an uphill struggle up the never-ending north face of Mount Crap, as I discover, thanks to life-long learning, new and exciting forms of crap piled on the old. And the *really* galling thing is how much of this faeculent matter is generated by bloody doctors, not bureaucrats. I mean, these bloody "quality care" sacred cows...'

'Tell me about it,' I said, hoping he wouldn't. Unfortunately, he didn't take the hint.

'This morning,' he said, 'I had a consultation with an asthmatic. The poor bloke had gone through the rigmarole of phoning up, booking an appointment, taking time off work and sitting in our waiting room, next to all the coughing, wheezing viral sponges, just because our "quality" repeat prescribing system recalled him. For *what*? A consultation which was basically, "How's it going?" / "Fine, thanks." I gave him a peak flow test to pad things out, but I don't care what the NSFs or the Clinical Governance Gestapo say, it was an outrageous waste of my time, and his.'

The Senior Partner took a swig of his ale, and stared into the glass.

'I will enumerate my objections,' he said. This was my cue to get another round in, quick. It was obviously going to be a long night. 'First, most treatment reviews are unnecessary. Why do I need to check a thyroxine or analgesia regime annually? Can't we rely on the punters to let us know if there's a problem? They already have a fairly low threshold for attending and they really don't need any more encouragement from me.

'Second, patients can usually monitor their own diseases these days: they have peak flow meters, BP monitors, pharmacy-based cholesterol tests and so on. We're potentially redundant, which can't come a moment too soon for me.

'Third, treatment reviews inevitably create work. Nine times out of ten, people who come in for clinical reviews always find something else to bloody mention while they're there. I don't actually blame them – who's going to make the effort to come in to the surgery just to have their repeat prescription card rubber-stamped? So a "Therapy Update" turns into a "While I'm here", and more time is wasted.

'And fourth, this is a classic case of doctors over-valuing illness. When will we learn that diseases like asthma or hypertension aren't as important to people as we'd like to believe, not when there's shopping to be done, giros to collect, cars to nick and so on? It's absurd expecting patients to take time off from their busy schedules just so that we can pretend we're providing a quality service. We should realign our values with the punters – in other words, we should care less. I mean to say, the only patients who attend religiously for treatment reviews are the obsessive basket cases who bring a year's worth of computer print-outs depicting their twice daily peak flow readings and these people shouldn't be encouraged to get to the doctor, they should be encouraged to get a life.'

'You forgot the fifth point,' I said. 'Treatment review consultations are bloody boring. Which is why I usually delegate them to Nurse Susie.'

JARGON

AS MUST BE clear by now, the NHS is a world-leader in jargon creation, and there isn't the space, or the will, for me to explain it all here. Some things are in the glossary at the end of the book, others you'll have to Google or have a guess at, but here's a rough translation of what the SP is on about in the passage above.

'Life-long learning', part of the 'Working Together, Learning Together' 'framework' introduced in 2001, is the result of a truly brilliant epiphany experienced by someone in an office somewhere. In a moment of genius, he or she realised that medicine is constantly evolving and doctors ought to ensure that they keep on top of this. Thank God s/he did so, because prior to that, everyone I knew was obviously relying on what they learned in medical school 30 years ago.

'Quality care' is another similar load of guff which is supposed to 'put quality at the heart of the NHS' but, as the Senior Partner is discovering, often has exactly the opposite effect.

'NSFs' (National Service Frameworks) are a set of dictatorial rules imposed on a group of people in surgeries who know what they're doing by a group of people in offices who don't know what they're doing.

The 'Clinical Governance Gestapo' are the people who check up on you to make sure you're doing these unnecessary things.

TRACEY'S RASH JUDGMENT

I COULD TELL Tracey was trouble from the moment she walked in.

She was straight out of the *Fat Slags*: leggings, a tight white top that barely contained her fulsome person and an expression somewhere between rage and disbelief.

She sat down and started gabbling at 90 miles per hour.

'So I've got this rash, yeah? So I seen that Dr Gavin about it…'

'Gavin Hall? He's actually a locum, but carry on.'

'What? He ain't even a real doctor?'

'No, a locum is… look, we trust him on rashes.'

'Whatever.' She hoiked up her top: there was, indeed, a red smear across her midriff. 'So I seen him, right, and he just calls it a fancy name and says it's nuffink serious, yeah? I mean, look at that! Nuffink serious?! He says if it itches to rub some of that Caroline lotion in…'

'Calamine?'

'Whatever. To rub some of that in if it itches, and otherwise it'll just go away of its own afford. So I says to him, I ain't being funny, yeah, but I'm going to Jamaica for Christmas in three bleeding weeks and I ain't going looking like this. So he says, "Well, I'm sorry, madam, right, but there's really nuffink else I can do, yeah?" So I said I wanted someone else to have a look, which is why I'm here.'

'Oh dear.'

I really dislike having to provide an instant 'second opinion' for disgruntled punters with minor ailments. It puts me in an impossible situation. I'm sure that Gavin will have examined Tracey far more meticulously than I would have bothered to, and will have spent precious NHS time explaining the likely benign nature of her problem before advising her down the calamine lotion route. The truth is, there's probably nothing else *I* can do, either. But people like Tracey don't want the truth.

As she carried on yattering away, I turned over the possibilities in my mind.

Scenario A (most likely): Gavin's assessment is perfectly accurate. It's Pityriasis rosea, and it really is nothing to worry about. As far as we know, it's a viral infection producing a characteristic skin eruption that fades after six weeks or so, and you're unlikely to get it again.

Scenario B (not impossible): Gavin has done all the right things but has diagnosed as viral Pityriasis rosea a rash which to my slightly more experienced eye looks more typical of a fungal skin infection called Pityriasis versicolor. An easy mistake to make that leaves me with a dilemma: P. rosea will burn itself out; P. versicolor won't. In fact, it will become even more apparent in sun. If my hunch is right, and Tracey wants to look good on the beach, she ought to be using antifungal treatment from tomorrow.

If I stick up for Gavin and it turns out he was right, great.

If I stick up for him and it turns out he was mistaken, it makes us both look stupid.

If I say that he might be wrong and offer an alternative diagnosis, that makes him look stupid and me a smart arse.

And if I say that he was wrong and it turns out that he was right, I'm the berk who prescribed an unnecessary antifungal treatment.

Time for the 'lab test as delaying tactic' approach.

'Tracey, it's almost certain that Dr Hall is correct but if you'd like me to organise a couple of investigations... perhaps I could take some skin scrapings from the rash?'

Moments later, and after some self-righteous harrumphing, she was happily queuing for a blood test with the practice nurse.

Which was when I heard another eruption, this time more volcanic than cutaneous, as she deciphered my handwriting on the request form: 'Rash of unknown cause. Possible secondary syphylis.'

Ah yes, Scenario C. Perhaps I should have mentioned that earlier.

HOW TO SAVE THE NHS BILLIONS WITHOUT ANYONE NOTICING

I'M NOT USUALLY one to agree with management consultants, but they recently suggested the NHS workforce should be cut by 10% to save money. This surely merits further consideration. In fact, I'd like to make some suggestions of my own about NHS staff who we could sack tomorrow and who wouldn't exactly be sorely missed – largely because we wouldn't notice, or care:

Health visitors: they're supposed to have a 'special role' in the care of new mothers and new babies. It's so special, in fact, that no one really knows what it is. What I do know is that they create unnecessary anxiety in parents by suggesting that an umbilical polyp might be something rare and serious (wrong and wrong) or unnecessary work for me by misdiagnosing sticky eye as conjunctivitis and sending mother/child to my emergency clinic.

Counsellors: 'talking treatments' are seen as a panacea these days. In a way, they are – for the GP rather than the patient. Because they enable us to tell the emotionally incontinent to go away, but nicely. Like the rest of us, counsellors are 70% water; unlike the rest of us, the other 30% is fluff. I believe they make good tea, though.

Anyone involved with: Choose and Book, Referral Management Centres, NHS Direct and the Summary Care Record: all obscene wastes of time and money.

Pre-op assessment nurses: these are nurses who check you over before you have surgery. All they do is measure your blood pressure and dipstick your urine, yet they manage to screw both up. A slight blip in your BP when they've just outlined the possible complications of your op (eg death) does not constitute hypertension, it constitutes being scared. And minor abnormalities in your wee are of no interest to anyone, least of all me. Yet somehow these irrelevances might lead to the cancellation of your surgery until I 'sort it all out'.

Psychiatrists: 'Dear Dr Copperfield, your patient did not attend clinic today, so I've discharged him from the mental health services back to your care.' Fantastic – never mind he DNA'd because he's convinced you're working for the CIA and is therefore more in need of shrink-care than ever. I'd suggest it was a way of massaging the waiting lists if I didn't think it would get me sectioned for being paranoid.

Physiotherapists who have bestowed on them the epithet 'practitioner', as in 'upper limb practitioner', 'lower limb practitioner', 'left middle finger practitioner' and so on. I realise I've gone on about this elsewhere, but it bears repetition. I want an orthopaedic opinion, so I refer the patient for one. But my referral is 'managed' in the direction of some middle tier quasi-service, with the result that I get a letter from a jumped-up physio who makes some dumb-ass suggestions and who, nine months and no progress later, suggests I refer the patient for an orthopaedic opinion. Brilliant.

Noctors: a Noctor is a 'nurse practitioner' who patients incorrectly assume is a doctor. They are increasingly used as an intermediary between myself and the specialist I really wanted you to see. For more details, see 'physiotherapist practitioner', above.

Anyone from the PCT who writes letters describing their 'vision' of primary care, who uses the word 'robust' whenever they can't think of another adjective or who describes primary care as trying to create a 'virtuous circle, with the patient in the middle': yes, really.

Social workers: OK, I realise that, strictly speaking, they don't work for the NHS, but I thought it unfair to leave them out.

Management consultants: what the hell do they know?

THAT WILL TEACH ME

THEY SAY THE greatest feeling in medicine is healing the sick, but they're wrong.

The greatest feeling in medicine is healing the last sick person of the day and then closing the surgery door behind you with a clunk.

Mr Bell was the final patient of my emergency surgery. Chelsea were about to take on Liverpool in the Premiership, and while I didn't have a dog in the fight I *did* have a beer in the fridge, a telly with surround sound and a wife who was away at her mum's.

Mr Bell was getting a script for amoxicillin regardless, and then I was out of there.

The first thing I noticed was the lop-sided smirk on his face. *Probably a TATT who's sneaked in through the back door and realises he has me at his mercy*, I thought.

'It's my bloody face, doc,' he said, drooling slightly as he spoke. 'It started two or three days ago.'

So the grin was involuntary. Blimey: a unilateral facial paralysis. I checked him out. No other neurological symptoms. Ears and parotid OK[1]. Bingo.

'You've got Bell's Palsy,' I said. 'Which is ironic, given your name. I haven't seen one for ages. No-one knows what causes it, but it's not usually a major problem – most cases clear up OK in a few weeks.'

'What's the treatment, doc?' he said.

'Hmmm,' I said. 'Good question. Some doctors reckon steroids help. Some don't. And I...err...don't. Don't know, that is. They're not essential. How are you about taking pills?'

'I'm not that keen, to be fair.'

'OK, that's settled, then. Make an appointment for a week from now and we'll have another gander at you.'

By which time, hopefully, you'll be looking a bit less creepy.

He left happy, and I was happier still. Bag shut. Desk cleared. Then guilt and diligence kicked in. I looked at my watch: still plenty of time to get home for kick-off. I switched my PC back on, got onto google and, in 30 seconds, I was confronted by more than I ever wanted to know about Bell's Palsy. And, sodding hell: 'Steroids and aciclovir [an anti-viral drug] increase complete resolution rates from 80% to 97%'.[2]

What? Why didn't anyone tell me? Bugger.

It got worse: 'Gold standard treatment... most effective if started within three days of onset...'

I looked at my watch again. I had... let's see ...half an hour. Bloody hell.

I phoned Mr Bell's home number. Engaged. Try again. Engaged. Phone phone phone. Engaged engaged engaged.

Bugger. Bugger. Bugger.

I was going to have to call in on my way home. No problem. I might miss the first five minutes of the match, but the opening exchanges are likely to be cagey.

I checked the route. Holy cow! Mr Bell's address wasn't on the map – it was on some poxy new estate. I started developing a tension headache.

My mind flitted to Dr Emma. Only the day before, I'd asked her why she looked like death-warmed-up.

'No sleep last night,' she said. It transpired she'd developed an acute anxiety state about a patient she'd seen – a baby with D&V who she'd decided, retrospectively, was borderline dehydrated and therefore needed follow-up. So she rang – no answer. She visited – no reply. She called A&E and the paediatric unit – no joy. Which meant a night awake imagining expiring babies, distraught parents and terminated careers. She visited next morning before breakfast. Of course, everything was fine – they'd just spent the evening at granny's.

I groaned. Deep down, no matter how burnt out or cynical we appear, we do care. The root of this caring may be vocational, professional, medicolegal, or all three, but it's real.

In the end, the police directed me to Mr Bell and his Palsy. He decided that he would take the acyclovir and prednisolone, and that I was a very caring doctor.

By then it was half time and I had missed two goals and 45 minutes of the match of the season.

I can smile about it now, though. And so can he.

[1] A patient with a serious ear infection may rarely develop facial paralysis. The parotid is the largest salivary gland; tumours in this gland can also cause facial paralysis.

[2] Since writing this piece, the powers-that-be have decided that patients with Bell's probably *don't* need aciclovir after all because, 'A randomised trial showed that… blah blah blah.'

Like I say, it's a bugger.

MR NICKLEBY REDUX

I GOT A CHRISTMAS card in my pigeon hole today from Mr Nickleby's family.

It thanked me for what I'd done for him over the years and contained a note he'd written before he died and which, apparently, he'd asked to be passed on to me.

All it said was: 'I knew there was something wrong.'

Mr Nicklebys come and Mr Nicklebys go, and it's at times like this that you wonder whether the feelings you harbour are guilty relief or perverse sadness; certainly in this case, I can't decide one way or the other. One thing's for sure, though: wherever he is now, I hope that buzzing in his ear has gone.

HAPPY CHRISTMAS, WAR IS OVER

I PULLED UP IN the surgery car park for my last working day of the year. Sami Patel had beaten me to the Senior Partner's space, so I nosed into the box marked 'Practice Manager'. I felt like the World's Strongest Man must feel after shedding himself of one of those unfeasibly large boulders: for once, I'd wangled some time off over the festive period, and the opportunity to thumb my nose at authority was the icing on my plum duff.

Unfortunately, Jane Carstone had followed me in, so after getting out of my car I sheepishly got back into it and re-parked in the nurse's space. Jane actually smiled at me and mouthed 'Thank you', so I decided to wait while she got out of her BMW.

'Morning,' I said. 'Sorry about the parking, but I didn't…'

'Oh, don't worry, Tony,' she said. 'Thank *you* for moving for me.'

We walked together to the surgery doors. Nemesis had returned with his indelible silver pen and a message for his hubristic rival:

Kyle Chuzzlewit is deffinitly a gayboy, everbody nos that

'I thought you were going to scrub all that off?' said Jane.

'I never got round to it,' I said. 'Maybe next year.'

'You could do it tomorrow,' said Jane. 'Didn't you get my message? We had to rejig the rota and you're in for the rest of the week.'

She walked in through the door, just as the sleet started.

I laughed, bitterly, and followed her.

Inside, all was tinsel and santa hats. Medically-speaking, the usual Christmas identifiers were present, too.

At the start of December, 90% of my chronic disease management mysteriously evaporates. The diabetic clinic empties. Obsessive cholesterol checkers vanish. The need for smoking cessation advice ceases.

It could be that these patients go AWOL because they know the Christmas party season screws up their sugars, lipid levels and smoking intentions. Or it might be that they simply have better things to do, so the symptom list is ditched in favour of the shopping list.

But the door marked 'GP' is a revolving one, so one group of patients is simply replaced by another – in this case, those for whom Christmas warps illness, behaviour and logic.

First up I was consulted by an apparently sensible woman with a cold who justified her attendance with the words: 'I don't want to be ill for Christmas.'

You don't say?

'I know you don't usually give antibiotics,' she said, 'but I thought, in view of the time of year…'

She looked hopefully at me, as though I might don a Santa outfit, and pluck from my sack a gift-wrapped bottle of pills. Maybe she genuinely believed that the biology of viruses changes in the presence of tinsel, leaving them suddenly susceptible to the amoxicillin they laugh at for the other 360-odd days of the year.

Either way, she was wrong, and out she flounced, muttering something about Scrooge.

The next contestant was a wilfully doleful young male – one of many patients who rarely darken my door except at the beginning of the festive season, at which time they appear and make pathetic attempts to extract a sick note.

'I think I might have flu,' he said, affecting a bit of a croak. 'I reckon I need a note, doc. No way can I go into work like this.'

'Out late last night, were we?' I said.

'I might have had a few,' he admitted. 'But this is no hangover, trust me.'

'Of course not,' I said. 'But it's not flu, either. Take a couple of paracetamol, drink plenty of water and you'll be right as rain. Next!'

Other attenders at the Christmas Cracker Clinic were more entertaining.

Towards the end of the afternoon, a young lady in a low-cut LBD and a hundredweight of make-up dropped in on her way to a party to check whether it was OK to drink alcohol with the anti-depressants she was taking for seasonal affective disorder (making me question just how SAD she actually was), and a middle-aged diabetic wanted to know if the season's goodwill extended to relaxing the NHS Viagra prescription rules. Sadly not, Casanova.

The final patient of the day was a young man who had photocopied his buttocks at the previous night's office do.

'I know it's mad, doctor,' he said, plaintively, 'but my mate reckons that the light from the copier is radioactive. What I want to know is, have I done any harm?'

'If you mean to your arse, no,' I said. 'Your career prospects are another thing altogether.'

You'd think that was unbeatable. Yet Sami Patel collared me in the car park.

'Oi, Copperfield,' he said, almost beside himself in his keenness to grab me. 'You won't believe this one... this patient has just texted us a photo of his backside, asking if I think it looks odd. He's worried he might have cancer. Er... piles, *maybe*. Anyway, guess what I emailed back?'

'Er...' I said. 'Something about a bum note?'

'No,' roared Sami. 'Is that the best you can do? No, I sent back, "Happy Christmas, Mr Jinkins. Nothing to worry about – I think it's just a problem with your ring tone." Geddit? *Ring tone*. He emailed it from his mobile and it was a picture of...'

I got into my Nissan and drove away, leaving Dr Patel standing in the car park cackling to himself.

BED BLOCKERS, BAPS AND BUFFING: A BLUFFERS GUIDE TO MEDICINE

AS PEOPLE DO in every other job, medics use abbreviations, euphemisms and jargon.

Some consultants are unwilling to utter the word 'cancer' in front of a patient, and will instead talk about 'large bowel lesions' and 'metastatic disease' in an effort to spare their feelings, before asking them to pop a sample of their 'Number Twos' into a specimen pot.

Then there are 'Three Letter Acronyms', usually abbreviated to the three letter acronym 'TLA', that refer to medical tests ('ECG') or common diagnoses ('IBS') and which save doctors and their secretaries hours of typing. These are fine when used within a particular speciality but cause havoc when they appear in letters to GPs. Mrs Squeers may well have had an ABG in Outpatients last week, but was that a measurement of her Arterial Blood Gases by a chest specialist or an Autologous Bone Graft at the hands of an orthopaedic surgeon?

Finally, there are the frequently derogatory terms that fly back and forth across A&E departments, GPs' coffee rooms and hospital wards.

These aren't usually written down, especially as modern computerised record systems don't allow much free texting and there is no 'ICD-10' code (see below) for, for example, 'Status Hispanicus'.

The selection that follows includes some very commonly used examples of MedSpeak, some less common and some that are, hopefully, apocryphal. Some are in the book, some aren't – some might be in your own medical notes, others might not.

A&E

Accident & Emergency – often re-jigged as 'Always and Everybody' to emphasise the 24/7 open access they offer.

Ash Cash

Payment to doctors for completion of the paperwork involved in organising a cremation.

BAPS

British Association of Plastic Surgeons. (How naïve are they?)

BChir or BCh

Baccalaureus Chirurgiæ (Bachelor of Surgery) – one of the two basic doctors' qualifications when obtained from a college that still thinks speaking in Latin is cool. English speakers tend to use B.S. (Bachelor of Surgery).

Bed blocker

A patient (often 'crumble' q.v.) stuck in an acute hospital bed they don't actually need, simply because there are no long term beds or nursing home placements available for them to transfer to.

BJGP

British Journal Of General Practice. A monthly publication where GPs who wear sports jackets without irony pontificate about 'holistic care' and the patient's 'inner journey'. Substantial contributions from GPs in the Netherlands, where strong lager and psychoactive drugs are widely available, add to the otherworldly nature of the journal.

BMA

British Medical Association. The doctors' professional body, and the nearest thing we have to a trade union. The BMA doesn't register or regulate the profession (c.f. GMC) but it negotiates with the Department of Health on our behalf and, as far as the media is concerned, is the doctors' mouthpiece.

BMJ

Previously known as the British Medical Journal. A weekly comic that includes details of recent original research, editorials summarising current medical treatments and job adverts. By all accounts the best of its type.

BNF

British National Formulary – a twice yearly publication that contains details of uses, doses and side effects of all currently available medicines. Invaluable and generally referred to as the doctors' 'prescribing bible'.

Bounceback

A patient who has been discharged from hospital prematurely and who requires re-admission (organised by the GP more often than not) for the same problem.

BP

Blood pressure, or British Pharmacopoeia, as in 'Pholcodine linctus, BP'. Medicines labelled 'BP' are manufactured to recognised quality standards. The suffix does not imply that a medicine is actually safe or effective.

Buffing

A subtle and often retrospective rewriting of a patient's medical record intended to imply that the doctor who first assessed the patient had considered the eventual diagnosis, especially if the diagnosis turned out to be serious and/or life-threatening. For example, adding the words, 'No apparent neck stiffness, visible rash or problems with bright lights' to the admission note of a child who developed meningitis. Not strictly ethical.

CAM

Complementary and Alternative Medicine. Also the name of a prescription drug used in the 1960s and 1970s to treat childhood asthma. Neither is/was particularly effective.

CATT

Crisis Assessment and Treatment Team. Not intended to make a drama out of a mental health crisis, but often successful in inadvertently doing so. Theoretically, the gateway to in-patient care and facilitators of early discharge into the community. Or, to put that another way, they do all they can to stop patients from getting into psychiatric hospitals and then turf them out as soon as they can.

CBT (1)

Cognitive Behavioural Therapist. Somebody who believes

that the best way to treat a patient's depression is to get them to stop behaving as if they're depressed. How about we try that with diabetes?

CBT (2)

Clot in a bow tie – derogatory term for hospital consultant used by angry GPs. Very angry GPs sometime resort to the alternative, c**t in a bow tie.

CFS

Chronic Fatigue Syndrome. The new and much preferred term for 'ME/Yuppie Flu/Postviral Fatigue Syndrome'.

CME

Continuing Medical Education. The requirement for doctors to attend promotional lectures while eating curry or stale *vol-au-vents*, both sponsored by the manufacturer of a new wonder drug, in the name of education.

COPD

Chronic Obstructive Pulmonary Disease. The new name for COAD (Chronic Obstructive Airway Disease) which was the new name for Chronic Bronchitis and Emphysema etc etc. I believe they call this 'progress'.

CPA

Care Programme Approach. A system designed to ensure that all patients with significant mental health problems get all the support and help they need. Includes personalised care plans, risk assessments and a letter to the GP every six months to say that the patient hasn't shown up for their Care Plan meeting. If we happen to know where they are, could we pop in and make sure they're OK?

C(A)T scanning

Computerized (Axial) Tomography. Sequential X-rays fashioned by a computer into an anatomically accurate image.

Usually referred to as a CT scan, the term CAT scan is now reserved for the punchline of the well-worn 'Lab tests and cat scan' joke.

Crackerjack call

'It's Friday, it's five o'clock, it's… *vital* that something is done about something, *now*.' Something that usually involves psychiatry, geriatrics and incontinence. You will only understand the reference if you watched children's TV in the 1970s.

Crumble

Widely used in hospital to describe geriatric patients who aren't acutely ill but who are suffering as a result of old age and frailty.

DBI

Dirt bag index. A rough and ready estimation of the number of hours since a patient's last bath or shower, calculated by multiplying the number of tattoos by the number of missing teeth.

DH

Department of Health. Went to the expensive trouble of changing its name (headed notepaper and all) because doctors would deliberately pronounce the previous abbreviation, DoH, with a Homer Simpson voice (and often include the palm slap to the face to emphasise the point that they were dealing with idiots.)

DKDC

Don't know don't care. There comes a point, usually at the end of a 25-minute consultation with a heartsink patient about their peculiar aches and pains and their funny turns, when the doctor realises that he doesn't know what's causing them and has frankly given up trying to make sense of the story. A prescription for vitamin tablets often follows.

DLA

Disability Living Allowance. You have the symptoms, we fill out the form, we both get some money. Result!

DNA

As we have seen, not only deoxyribonucleic acid but also 'Did Not Attend' – the patients who book appointments, fail to show up and unwittingly keep GPs' clinics running on time.

DRCOG

Diploma of the Royal College of Obstetricians and Gynaecologists. Most GPs have this postgraduate qualification.

DRT

Died right there. Paramedical term for a sudden unexpected death.

DRT, T, T & T

Died right there, there, there and there. Paramedical term for a violent death.

DSB

Drug-seeking behaviour. Exaggerating the severity of a painful symptom and casually mentioning the name of the patient's preferred medicine in an effort to secure a prescription for a codeine- or morphine-based painkiller or a Valium-like tranquilliser. Variants include ONDSB & OWDSB – 'Oscar-nominated' and 'Oscar-winning', respectively.

DSH

Deliberate Self Harm – self mutilation and head-banging that falls short of actual suicide.

DV

Domiciliary Visit. Rarer now than they were, a system that allows consultants (usually geriatricians and psychiatrists) to visit patients in their own home.

DWP

Department of Work and Pensions. To whom patients forward their sick notes to claim benefit. Famous for writing to patients on Tuesday to remind them that their last sick note ran out the previous Thursday. This causes no inconvenience to the patient or their doctor. Really, none at all.

EBM

Evidence-Based Medicine – the frankly ludicrous (if you're a complementary therapist) notion that medicine should be based on logic, reason, experiment and scientific principles.

ECG

Electrocardiogram – that thing where they connect wires to your wrists and ankles to check the workings of the heart.

ECT

Electro-Convulsive Therapy. That thing where they connect wires to patients' temples and throw the mains switch for a second or two until they pull themselves together.

EEG

Electroencephalogram. Similar, but this time we're monitoring the brain's activity rather than trying to erase all trace of it.

EMI

Elderly Mentally Ill. The new name for psycho-geriatrics, popular as it's so much easier to spell.

Fishing trip (aka Shotgunning)

Ordering dozens of tests in the hope that one of them will throw up a diagnosis. Popular with American doctors and recently-qualified UK graduates who are no longer taught how to examine or take a history from their patients.

FP10

NHS prescription form.

FRCS

Fellow of the Royal College of Surgeons. A surgeon who has passed enough exams to be appointed consultant, and who then gets to call himself 'Mr' (or 'Mrs'/'Miss' in the case of female docs) again, just to confuse the patients.

GMC

General Medical Council – the doctors' regulatory body who maintain the Register (from which substandard docs might be struck off) and who are in charge of doctors' revalidation in the post-Shipman era.

GP

General Practitioner (family doctor). Me.

Granny stacker

A multi-storey storage facility for elderly patients.

Handbag positive

Descriptive term used in A&E for an elderly and usually confused female patient who is sitting up on a hospital trolley clutching her handbag.

IBD

Inflammatory bowel disease. The serious stuff like Crohn's disease and ulcerative colitis.

IBS

Irritable bowel syndrome. The not so serious stuff like constipation, bloating and tummy cramps.

ICD-10

International Classification of Diseases 10. The list of diagnoses that IT programmers use to set up medical computer systems.

LOLINAD

As above, a Little Old Lady in No Apparent Distress – i.e. not in pain, not short of breath, not overly anxious. Used in A&E records when the cause for attendance isn't clear.

MB

Bachelor of Medicine. Medicinæ Baccalaureus for the pretentious.

MDT

Multi-disciplinary Teams. Motley crews made up of a doctor (usually) and a selection of paramedical staff.

MRCGP

Member of the Royal College of General Practitioners. A postgraduate qualification in General Practice, these days mandatory for any new GP.

MRI

Magnetic resonance imaging. Really fancy imaging technique that has superseded CT scanning in the 'I want a test and I want it now!' scenario.

NAD

Test result – officially, 'Nothing Abnormal Detected', occasionally, 'Never Actually Done'.

NFN

'Normal for Norfolk'. A clinical sign (classically an extra digit on either hand) that implies a degree of inbreeding. Often accompanied by 'JLD' – Just Like Dad – especially in WLK (q.v.) situations.

NICE

National Institute for Clinical Excellence.

OCD

Obsessive Compulsive Disorder. Look it up on Wikipedia. Then check to make sure you got it right. Then check again. One more check wouldn't hurt. And another, just to be on the safe side. Are you sure? Better check again. Are you certain it hasn't changed since last time you looked? How would you know? One last look and then it's time to go out. OK, just one more. Repeat *ad infinitum*.

OD

Overdose – or far more likely, underdose. If you find yourself being carefully coached about the minimum lethal dose of paracetamol and alcohol by a harassed on-call psychiatrist, rest assured that he's starting to tire of meeting up with you in A&E every time your boyfriend/girlfriend/mum/dad annoy you.

OT

Occupational Therapist. A person whose occupation is 'therapist'.

PALS

Patient Advice & Liaison Service. The hospital department I will advise you to contact when Outpatient services let you down, rather than let you bitch to me about it.

Parentectomy

Admitting a child to hospital simply to separate the poor kid from its panicking/negligent/NFN parents for a period of respite.

PCT

Primary Care Trust.

PDP

Personal Development Plan. This is what I'm supposed to generate, maintain and review at regular intervals. What I'm supposed to develop into has never been made clear.

PFO

Pissed, fell over. Commonly (very, very commonly) used A&E abbreviation.

PGT

Pissed, got thumped. Commonly (very, very commonly) used A&E abbreviation.

Pt c/o

The first symptom the patient mentions, occasionally the one they're really bothered about: Patient complaining of X.

Pumpkin sign

Another A&E record entry implying that shining a pen torch in to the patient's mouth would illuminate the entire head like a Halloween pumpkin. Implies an element of oligo-neurality. (Oligo = not many; neurones = brain cells.)

PUNs & DENs

As discussed earlier, PUNs are 'Patients' Unmet Needs' and DENs are 'Doctors' Educational Needs'. Not only are we expected to find out what patients really want and, if necessary, look stuff up in textbooks to find the answers for them, we're also expected to write little essays about the experience in our spare time. A big, big favourite with GPs who wear cardigans.

QALY

Quality Adjusted Life Year. Enables health economists to decide whether it's worth spending any more public money keeping you alive.

QOF

The fabulous Quality & Outcomes Framework.

Status Hispanicus

A play on 'status epilepticus' – an ongoing and uncontrollable epileptic fit. SH refers to patients who scream and gesticulate wildly about the unbearable nature of their symptom (usually pain and or weakness) without conveying any information that might actually help their doctor make a diagnosis. For example, 'Where does it hurt?' 'Everywhere!' 'How long has it been troubling you? 'Forever!' etc. etc. Apologies to non-hysterical Hispanic readers.

Syndrome detector

Inbuilt diagnostic feature possessed by good doctors. Kick-started by the feeling that something just ain't right with a patient, it enables the doctor to assemble a selection of apparently disconnected individual symptoms into one recognisable whole, a syndrome.

TEETH

Tried Everything Else, Try Homoeopathy.

TTFO

According to legend, one quick-thinking doctor quizzed by a judge about the meaning of this entry in a medical record explained that it meant 'Told Take Fluids Orally'.

Turfing

The process of shifting a time-consuming patient from one discipline or doctor to another. Surgeons will turf a patient with recurring abdominal pain to the physicians if there's no need for an urgent operation, the physicians will turf him on to the geriatricians as he's over 60 years old and they will, in turn, turf him back to the GP to organise investigations as an outpatient.

WLK

Weird Looking Kid – aka 'FLK' for 'funny-looking kid': a child that might trigger a doctor's Syndrome Detector (q.v.) leading to investigations that simply prove that he's NFN and JLD. Occasionally – very, very occasionally – accompanied by GLM.

Second Opinion: A Doctor's Dispatches from the Inner City
Theodore Dalrymple (hdbk, £14.99)

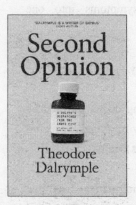

No-one has travelled further into the dark and secret heart of Britain's underclass than the brilliant Theodore Dalrymple. A hospital consultant and prison doctor in the grim inner city, every day he confronts a brutal, tragic netherworld which most of us never see. It's the world of 'Baby P' and Shannon Matthews, where life is cheap and ugly, jealous men beat and strangle their women and 'anyone will do anything for ten bags of brown'. In a series of short and gripping pieces, full of feeling and bleak humour, he exposes the fascinating, hidden horror of our modern slums as never before.

'Dalrymple's dispatches from the frontline have a tone and a quality entirely their own... their rarity makes you sit up and take notice'
– Marcus Berkmann, The Spectator

'Dalrymple is a modern master'
– Stephen Poole, The Guardian

'The George Orwell of our time... a writer of genius'
– Denis Dutton

**From all good bookshops, online from
www.mondaybooks.com or via 01455 221752.**

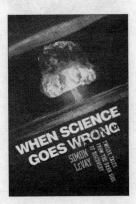

Perverting The Course Of Justice / Inspector Gadget
(ppbk, £7.99)

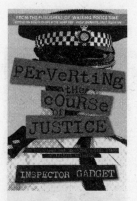

A senior serving policeman picks up where PC Copperfield left off and reveals how far the insanity extends – children arrested for stealing sweets from each other while serious criminals go about their business unmolested.

'Exposes the reality of life at the sharp end'
– *The Daily Telegraph*

'No wonder they call us Plods... A frustrated inspector speaks out on the madness of modern policing'
– *The Daily Mail*

'Staggering... exposes the bloated bureaucracy that is crushing Britain' – *The Daily Express*

'You must buy this book... it is a fascinating insight'
– Kelvin MacKenzie, *The Sun*

A Paramedic's Diary / Stuart Gray
(ppbk, £7.99)

STUART GRAY is a paramedic dealing with the worst life can throw at him. *A Paramedic's Diary* is his gripping, blow-by-blow account of a year on the streets – 12 rollercoaster months of enormous highs and tragic lows. One day he'll save a young mother's life as she gives birth, the next he might watch a young girl die on the tarmac in front of him after a hit-and-run. A gripping, entertaining and often amusing read by a talented new writer.

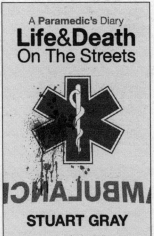

As heard on BBC Radio 4's Saturday Live and BBC Radio 5 Live's Donal McIntyre Show and Simon Mayo

In April 2010, Stuart Gray was named one of the country's 'best 40 bloggers' by *The Times*

From all good bookshops, online from www.mondaybooks.com or via 01455 221752.

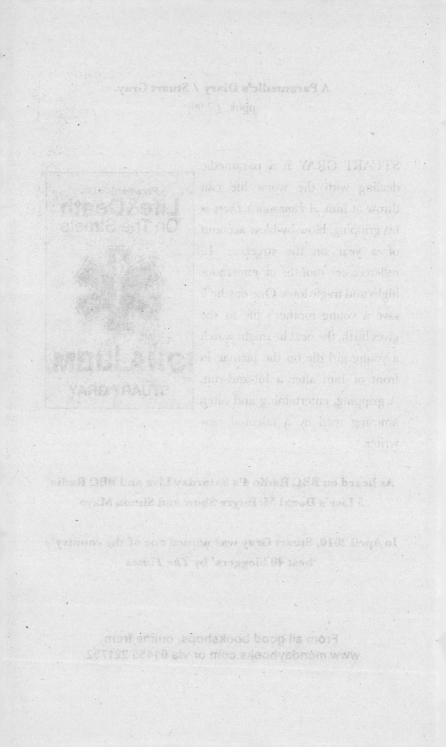